Never Enough Nation

Managing Your Health, Wealth, and Stress

Never Enough Nation

Managing Your Health, Wealth, and Stress

By

Jeff Gaines and Jim Sorensen

Never Enough Nation
Managing Your Health, Wealth and Stress

Cover Design by Brian Golden

ISBN-10: 0-61569-355-5

ISBN-13: 978-0-61569-355-2

Book Website: NeverEnoughNation.com

Printed in the USA by Create Space

To the love of my life, Noel

To my pride and joy, Aiden

And to Mom, Dad, and Bill

JDG

To my Mom, Brenda, and Katelyn:

the three women who helped me see that I am enough.

JMS

Table of Contents

Part Three
Winning the Game

Appendix

Acknowledgements

Jeff Gaines

I first want to thank my co-author, Jim Sorensen. I am the voice you will hear throughout this book. Jim has contributed greatly to the content and collaborated on the rest. This book would not be what it is without him and those who know him will hear his voice in many places.

I also want to thank Dana Bennett, Mary Judd, and especially Goody Niosi for their editing contributions.

Lastly, my thanks to the following for their commentary, critique, and support. Their honest feedback and selfless contribution of time helped lift this book to a whole different level: Doug Cellineri, Matthew Fairfax, Antoinette Perez, Sarah Richey, and of course, Brenda Sorensen and Noel Gaines.

Jim Sorensen

I want to thank Jeff for all the work he did and the tenacity it took to birth this book. It was a fun, insightful, and challenging collaboration.

I also want to thank the people who supported me early in my life to take the path of facilitation: Randy Revell, Pat Fandrich, and Robin Fitzgerald (now Lake). They each saw something in me I didn't see.

And lastly, and most notably, the two most important people in my life: my wife Brenda, the best thing that ever happened to me, and my daughter Katelyn, a gift to me in so many ways.

Introduction

The American culture is obsessed with having more of everything. This book is about feeling that what you *have* and who you *are* is enough. For anyone with the common perfectionist mindset, the words "good enough" feel like giving up. We are conditioned to believe that unless we are striving for and wanting more than what we have now, we are settling; we are giving less than our best. The goal of this book is for you to feel that you give your best AND that *who you are* and *what you have* is enough.

When someone can't feed their family, struggles to afford safe housing, can't afford to take their child to a doctor, battles serious health issues, etc., I think we can agree they don't have enough. This book is about why you might still feel that you don't have enough, even when you are well beyond the previous points.

How much of a burden is the Never Enough Mindset? I'll ask you to explore that question, but that's not to say that all your struggles come from not feeling like you have enough. That would be a gross oversimplification. There are many reasons why your physical health, financial health, and stress levels are the way they are, but I think most people reading this book will find that the Never Enough Mindset is a familiar part of their everyday life.

You've heard the expression, "It's not what you say, it's how you say it." I don't agree. It's not what you say, it's not even how you say it, it's *why* you say it. The *why* is the core intention that drives the "what" and the "how."

This is a good analogy for what this book is about because it is not a "how to" book. It will not tell you how to handle your money, exercise, eat right or manage your schedule. There are already a ton of great books that do that. This book is about why you don't read those books, or if you do, why you might struggle putting them into practice.

We are going to explore the *why* behind your health, wealth, and stress. When you know how to change that driving intention, the "what" and the "how" will look and feel different and be easier to master. Some of you might even find that you don't need to change the physical results of your life, you just need to change how you experience the life you already have, which also comes from the *why*.

Not All Struggles Are Created Equal

For most of the book, we are going to deal with health, wealth, and stress together because they all are driven by the same *why*. However, there is one major difference among the three. You don't have to spend money or over-schedule yourself, but you do have to eat. Plus, health is the only area of the three that has different genetic and biological factors. You can take two people and give them the exact same diet and amount of physical activity, and they won't necessarily display the exact same results.

Unfortunately, our society tends to see someone who is overweight as a lazy, gluttonous person lacking in self-control. In reality, they might be someone who actually has more self-control than the skinny person next to them. If their body is genetically more prone to fat storage than the skinnier person, they could be using significantly more discipline and self-control and still end up with a heavier body. Or, they could be experiencing a built-in higher degree of temptation, meaning they have more to overcome when battling temptations.

While most people who struggle with their weight do so because they eat more or worse food, and/or exercise less, it's not accurate to make this assumption for everyone. Plus, we are also going to find a biological link to why we struggle with wealth and stress. To put it another way, we all have our internal struggles, but they are not the same for all of us. Some people have a bigger fight due to the genetics of their brains and/or bodies.

> "This man beside us also has a hard fight with an unfavouring world, with strong temptations, with doubts and fears, with wounds of the past which have skinned over, but which smart when they are touched. It is a fact, however surprising. And when this occurs to us we are moved to deal kindly with him, to bid him be of good cheer, to let him understand that we are also fighting a battle; we are bound not to irritate him, nor press hardly upon him nor help his lower self". – John Watson (Ian MacLaren's real name) from "Courtesy", 1903.

None of us escapes this battle inside and few fully master it. I feel strongly that there are changes going on in our society, culture, and world that are driving our struggles with our health, wealth, and stress, and creating the Never Enough Nation.

Since we all have this fight inside us, it is a good idea to be kind to others who seem to be having a harder go of it. It is an even better idea to be kind to yourself. Most of us criticize ourselves mercilessly when we end up with a result we don't want. As it turns out, this doesn't make us better at correcting them, so let's stop and use education, support, and compassion instead. Enough is enough.

1

Temptations Running Amok

Do you have enough?

Some of you would say, "yes." But there can be a difference between what you believe and how you live. You might think you have enough, but do you live as though you do? If you spend more money than you make, eat more food than your body needs, and/or schedule a stress-filled, out-of-balance life, are you really living as though you have enough?

With more than sixty percent of Americans over-weight, over-spent or over-scheduled, most people don't live as though they have enough. It's not much of a stretch to call America the Never Enough Nation.

How much you are affected by the Never Enough Mindset is for you to decide. I ask you to keep an open mind from the start because the manner in which this mindset affects your thinking and behaviors can be subtle.

Where does the Never Enough Mindset come from?

Our ability to create temptations has exceeded our ability to resist them.

We are very good at making lots of yummy food, creating easy access to credit, and generating an endless variety of work, entertainment, and distractions to fill our schedules. Never in human history have we been surrounded by so much temptation: more, it seems, than we can control.

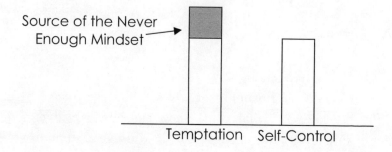

The Never Enough Mindset comes from the temptations that you just can't seem to satisfy, or you do so in unhealthy ways. If you don't satisfy a temptation, you end up feeling like you missed out and that your life may not be as good as it could have been. If you satisfy a temptation in a way that causes physical or emotional damage down the road, while you may have felt good in the moment, later you suffer guilt or shame and you end up feeling as if *you* are not enough. You lose either way. Suppress the temptation, or fulfill it in an unhealthy way, the end result is a feeling of not having enough or not being enough.

This Never Enough Mindset is sometimes hard to identify because you don't feel like you are sitting around "wanting" all the time. We rarely tell ourselves, "The problem with my life is that I just don't have enough." Instead, what we tell ourselves is, "I'm not happy with the results I'm getting. Why can't I get myself to do what I know I need to do to fix them?"

> ## We rarely notice the Never Enough Mindset; we feel the effects of it.

The effects of the Never Enough Mindset show up in our health, wealth, and stress levels. We are creating some very troubling results in these areas.

To summarize, the aim of this book is to help you manage your health, wealth, and stress. The problems you have in those areas often come from the Never Enough Mindset. The Never Enough Mindset comes from an excess of temptations that you try to suppress or satisfy in unhealthy or damaging ways. You'll have to either increase your self-control, or learn a better way to deal with your temptations.

The Solution

Most people buy into the belief that they just don't have enough will-power, meaning a lack of self-control is their problem. As it turns out, there are some things you can do to increase your self-control and we'll cover them, but these gains are usually modest. The better answer lies on the temptation side of the equation.

I don't think we are bad, weak-minded people who are just not strong enough to deal with our temptations. I think that because we live in such an amazing time and place, we have to develop skills that no nation in history has needed before. We simply have a level of temptation that those who came before us didn't have. As a result, we need skills they didn't need.

The solution is to learn how to *decrease* the temptation you experience. There are two ways to do this. The first method is to reduce or eliminate the temptations around you. You can do this using external methods, like getting rid of all the junk food in your house, or cutting up all your credit cards. You can also decrease the temptation you experience by changing how you see and react to the world around you. We will focus more on the latter, changing the inside, so that those temptations are just not as seductive.

The second way you can decrease the temptation you experience is to satisfy it. But often the problem is that the methods we use to satisfy our temptations create damage later. If you can satisfy your temptations in healthy and lasting ways, you will feel like you have enough.

The most effective strategy is going to be a combination of these approaches. I'm going to show you how to increase your self-control to the extent that you can, how to change the game on the inside, such that those temptations are just not as tempting, and how to satisfy your temptations in healthy and lasting ways.

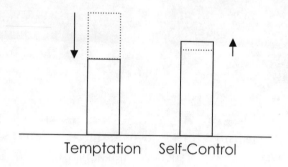

Temptation   Self-Control

This, by the way, is a great problem to have. We live in an amazing time and place. What we have is incredible. We just need to learn how to live with all this temptation without damaging ourselves. It's easier than you might think; we just don't have much education or practice doing it.

Our approach is going to be this:

Part One – The Internal Game

First, we need to learn about where temptation comes from. What are the internal mechanisms that drive temptation and self-control? We need to take a peek under the hood to better understand what makes us tick.

Part Two – The External Game

With a better understanding of how we operate, we'll go deeper into where all these temptations come from. What is going on in our society that is driving these out-of-control temptations? Plus, we'll go over some rules you can follow while interacting with the outside world that will make it easier for you to win the game.

Part Three – Winning the Game

You have deeply ingrained beliefs and behaviors. You've tried changing them with will-power, it usually doesn't work. With a deep understanding of what is going on inside you, clarity about how the outside world affects you, and some rules to follow, it will be time to put it all into action. Part three will show you what it really takes to make meaningful and lasting change in your life, and how to manage your wealth, health, and stress.

Part One

The Internal Game

2

Blame Your Brain

There is a game going on inside you every day. There are three players in this game and the field of play is your brain. Each of these players has their own special talents, strengths, and weaknesses. While there are things they do on their own, they rely heavily on each other.

The game they play is called the Internal Game. How this Internal Game plays out inside you has much to do with what happens outside you. That outside game is called the External Game.

Sometimes these players participate in the Internal Game as if they were highly skilled and well trained. Watching them play can be like watching a world class ballet, listening to a masterful orchestra or seeing your favorite sports team at its best. At other times it's like watching the Three Stooges.

Let's meet these players:

Player Profiles

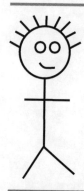

The Emoter

Strengths: Motivation, Persistence

Weaknesses: Cares Only About Right Now

Life's Purpose: Feel Good and Be Happy

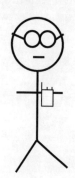

The Thinker

Strengths: Problem Solving, Critical
                        Thinking, Future Planning

Weaknesses: Short Endurance

Life's Purpose: Get the Emoter What it Wants

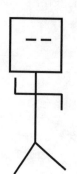

The Robot

Strengths: Memory, Performing
                        Repetitive Tasks

Weaknesses: Resistance to Change,
                        Limited by Past Experiences

Life's Purpose: Efficiency

Now let's watch the Internal Game in action.

(You get home after work and contemplate exercise.)

Emoter: Robot, look up exercise in the memory banks and tell me what you find.

Robot: Let's see, um, you hate it. Whining, crying, maybe some bleeding, not your favorite thing.

Emoter: Ick! I don't want to do that. Thinker, why on earth would we exercise?

Thinker: Well, turns out we have a high-school reunion coming up. Let's think about what it's going to be like walking in there.

Emoter: Double Ick! I don't want that. Thinker, come up with a way for us to not look like that at the reunion, *without* having to exercise.

Thinker: Well, we could not eat between now and then, but I'm going to recommend exercise anyway. But here's the thing: it's late, it's dark out, and there's a bunch of cars on the road. If we go for a walk, or run at this time of night, we might get hit by a car and die! It's a safety consideration. What we should do is get up an hour before work tomorrow and exercise then. The roads will be quiet and it will be a great start to our day.

Emoter: Great plan! What's on TV?

(Next day, an hour earlier than normal, the alarm goes off.)

Emoter: Oh, heck no! Thinker?

Thinker: We could exercise at lunch?

Emoter: Outstanding work! Snooze it is!

Does this conversation sound familiar to you? These players are always playing. The Internal Game goes non-stop. It shapes and informs your health, wealth, stress, and more. While this game plays out every day, all day, most people pay little attention to it.

These three separate, but interconnected drivers inside each of us compete for, and take turns choosing our actions. Not knowing that these players exist and not having any understanding about their strengths and weaknesses causes problems. You sometimes let the wrong player make your choices at the wrong time, and in the wrong way. Mastering your Internal Game is how you manage the Never Enough Mindset.

To understand these players, we need to start by looking at the *results* we produce. Where do our results come from? Behaviors. What we do gives us what we get.

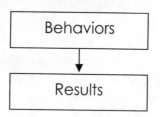

For example, if you call a friend and say, "I'm not happy with my job," what will they tell you? "Quit. You can do better than that." Same with a relationship. "If you are not happy with them, dump'em!" The basic approach being, if you are not happy with your results, change your behavior. Want to change your weight? Go on a diet, which is a new behavior plan. Want to change your financial health? Get on a budget, which is another new behavior plan. The advice for couples? Date night.

The same is true for organizations. Companies that are not getting the results they want implement new policies, new procedures, get new software systems, reorganize, upsize, downsize, rightsize, etc. We love these behavior modification programs. But according to a JD Powers study, sixty-five percent of corporate reorganizations fail to meet their stated objectives, so it usually doesn't work.

For most people, their "bag of tricks" for changing their ways begins and ends with behavior modification. Which is why, most of the time, they fail to create lasting change. Case in point: January in my gym. I hate January in my gym. Every year, my gym is swarmed by the New Year's Resolution crowd, huffing and wheezing up and down the court with their new shoes and shorts and creating long lines for equipment. By February, they've all quit and we can get back to life as usual.

Most people who go on a diet gain back the weight they lost, and then some. Most people who do debt consolidation end up deeper in debt, and the examples go on and on. Short term, will-power-based behavior modification almost never works, and that's probably not news to you. So why do people do it? Why are most of the books out there just another "behavior plan" that the reader won't stick to? Because it's all people know. If we want to get past behavior modification and will-power, we'll have to dig deeper.

Results come from behaviors, but where do behaviors come from? *Why* do we do what we do? The Thinker, Robot, and Emoter are the answer. Like passengers in a car, they take turns at the wheel. Each has their own agenda, interests, strengths, and weaknesses. The one in the driver's seat will determine the direction (behavior) we choose and the results we create.

The Internal Game

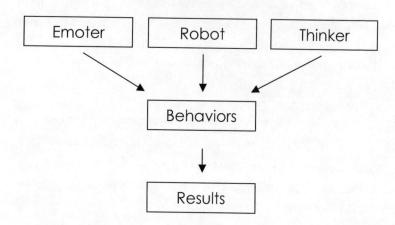

We make destructive choices because, most of the time, we let either the Emoter (emotions and feelings) or the Robot (past conditioning) call the shots, and put the Thinker (logic) in the backseat. In the areas of your life that are not working well, the Thinker rarely gets to drive. If the Emoter is not in charge, then it's the Robot that simply repeats the past behaviors it has learned from the Emoter, even if they don't work well. This pattern is usually the root cause of most of our problems.

All three affect the choices we make, but we have very little understanding, education or experience working with the three in unison. For the most part, people just think about the Thinker and believe it is in charge, when it is not. Only recently has the science community and, even more recently, the business world, seen any value in understanding how much the Emoter runs our lives.

We think we are logical creatures but all evidence shows that the contrary is true. How logical is it to be over-weight, over-spent or over-scheduled? How logical is war? How logical is a massive national debt, declining education system, etc? We are anything but a thinking species. The problem is we *think* we are. The good news is we can *learn* to be.

Revisiting the Never Enough Mindset

To review, the Never Enough Mindset comes from the temptations we experience that are beyond our ability to manage and moderate in healthy ways.

The Emoter is the origin of temptation because temptation is a wanting, yearning or longing. It is something we feel. The Thinker is our source of self-control. It is the area where our ability to reason, problem solve, determine the future impact of our actions, and moderate impulses manifest.

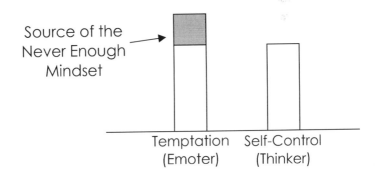

Source of the
Never Enough
Mindset

Temptation   Self-Control
(Emoter)   (Thinker)

You can see that the Never Enough Mindset comes from this internal struggle between your Emoter and your Thinker. You are tempted by what the Emoter thinks will make you happy. The Thinker knows better. We all know there is only so much the house, car, money, food, etc. can do to make us happy, but when the Emoter is behind the wheel, logic has little to do with it. When we put this equation in balance, the Thinker decides how to work effectively with the Emoter, rather than the Emoter deciding how to please itself. Alone, the Emoter doesn't make very good choices.

We humans continue to make less than healthy choices because we have a very limited understanding of our Emoters, our weak and underused Thinkers, and our poorly programmed Robots. In the following chapters we'll delve into each of these drivers to gain a deeper understanding of them. Then we will work on learning how to get the three to work together more effectively, creating the results we are after and, more importantly, feeling like those results are enough.

3

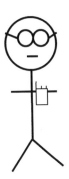

It's Elementary Watson!
The Thinker

The human forehead goes straight up, rather than sloping back like it does on other animals. This is because we have a piece of real estate in the front of our brains called the Frontal Lobes that contain a really interesting part named the Pre-Frontal Cortex. If you strip off this part of the human brain, the pieces you have left are roughly the same ones that Taco, our family dog's brain has. (Taco is a rescue dog from Mexico and my son Aiden wanted to name him after the Mexican word for a taco, so we did.)

The Pre-Frontal Cortex is the part of the brain where processes like problem solving, reasoning, and impulse control occur. We are going to call this function of the brain, the Thinker. If you take a teenager learning to drive a car and wire up their head so you can watch their brain process in real-time, their Pre-Frontal Cortex will be firing like crazy. They have to *think* their way through every step. If you were to look at the activity of your Pre-Frontal Cortex while driving, it would be void of activity. Have you ever arrived at your destination and asked yourself, "How did I get here?" Very complex thing driving, but your brain is programmed to do it without conscious thought. Your Robot does the driving and the Thinker is free to plan your weekend.

The Thinker is a vital and important part of your brain. In the words of Harvard psychologist Daniel Gilbert, author of *Stumbling on Happiness,* "The Pre-Frontal Cortex is what got us out of the cave and into the shopping mall." It is the source of all the amazing things humanity has accomplished. But because it is an add-on to the brain, a recent modification if you will, we are still very inexperienced in our use of it and have not yet mastered it.

The Long and The Short of it

Years ago, early in the development of this book, I called my co-author Jim, and asked him what he thought it takes to break habits. He said, "Basically, clear vision and good support." But then I said, "Wait a minute. *You* don't really use vision or goals, do you?" He laughed and said, "No." From my perspective, he just sort of wanders through life and always seems to end up in a better place than he was before, even when bad things happen. It's really very annoying.

When I probed further into Jim's amazingly deep yet very simple mind, he said, "When something comes along I ask myself, what is present reality and where will this take me? If it looks good, I do it." Further maddeningly annoying. After my years of research and endless contemplation, he summed it up, just that easily. What Jim has done is built a very strong and busy Thinker. The Emoter doesn't care about the future, only right now. The Thinker is the function in your brain that can use future consequences to drive decision making.

The Thinker is that part of your brain that can "see" the future. It is a big "what if" machine that can project a series of steps into the future and predict an outcome. Taco the dog doesn't have a Thinker. He acts on conditioning alone, without concern for future consequences. He sees the cat walk across the living room and the game is afoot! Off he goes, without regard to how much trouble he is going to get into.

Dog Internal Game

Robot: Cat.

Emoter: Run!

(Human: No! Bad dog!)

Emoter: I'm sorry. Please love and feed me.

We repeat bad habits because we act like Thinker-less dogs. We push aside or misuse the planning part of our brain and have our immediate desires drive our choices. We sort of de-evolve, if you will, to the point where we didn't have frontal lobes and just acted on impulse and conditioning. Try to explain to a four-year-old the concept of waiting and you'll understand what it is like to not have this ability. Children live in the present and have not yet developed the ability to plan out their actions, see the cause and effect of their choices, or understand that we are not going camping for three more weeks, so they might as well stop asking if we are going yet!

The Thinker is the only part of the brain that can use the future to drive our choices. Since most people have Thinkers that are underdeveloped to operate in the world that we live in today, the massive amount of emotional temptations around us overcharges our Emoters, which then overwhelm our Thinkers, and the future plays little role in our choices. The Thinker sees the long of it and the Emoter sees the short of it.

Active vs. Passive Thinker

For ease of understanding, we are going to refer to two modes that the Thinker operates in: Passive and Active. These are not meant to be literal definitions of the brain's functioning, so apologies to the scientific community. These two modes are analogies for the very different ways we use our Thinkers. Understanding these modes is going to be central to your success in getting the results you want.

Passive Thinker Mode

When in Passive mode, the Thinker is a servant to the other parts of your brain that contain the Emoter and the Robot. It is not running your decision-making; it is in support to either the Emoter or Robot, whichever is in charge. When the Robot is in charge, it is carrying out past programming, and when the Emoter is in charge, it is getting what it wants without regard for future consequences. The Passive Thinker is busy; it's just not in charge.

> **The primary job of a Passive Thinker is to satisfy the Emoter RIGHT NOW!**

A Passive Thinker Will Allow the Robot to go Un-Checked

One study says that for at least forty percent of your day, the Robot is in charge. I think it is more than that, but it's difficult to quantify. The Thinker has the ability to override the Robot and take charge but more often than not, we turn things over to the Robot. We'll learn more about why we do this in the Robot chapter, but for now we need to understand that the Thinker can take charge should we see fit, but in Passive mode, it does not.

The Thinker Can "Adjust Perceptions" to Help the Emoter Be Right

"Faced with the choice between changing one's mind and proving that there is no need to do so, almost everybody gets busy on the proof." - John Kenneth Galbraith

We all like to be right. Actually, the Emoter likes to be right. That makes sense, because being wrong doesn't *feel* good. Nobody wakes up in the morning with the thought, "You know what I'd like today? To be wrong." Unfortunately, sometimes life does not cooperate. When this happens, the Thinker gets to work finding ways to twist, distort, and warp what is going on around you to make the Emoter feel better.

Let's say you work with someone who you don't like, and they do something great. The Emoter feels very annoyed because there is evidence in front of it that contradicts its world view. This just won't do. So the Thinker, in Passive mode, goes to work to change your perception, rather than changing your belief. The Thinker starts making suggestions like, "It wasn't that big a deal, any moron could have done that." Or, "They probably took credit for someone else's work." Or, the Thinker will even start making things up like, "I bet they're embezzling." When acting as a servant to the Emoter, the Thinker can perform amazing feats of mental gymnastics to avoid having to change your mind and have the Emoter feel wrong.

The Passive Thinker Can Justify Almost Any Action

The Emoter likes to get what it wants, but sometimes you have to do some work to get what you want AND feel like it's okay to get it. When what you want is not the best choice for you in the future, your Thinker has some work to do. The Emoter cares about right now, so as long as the Thinker can find some logic, reasoning or justification to have the present action look good, the Emoter will be happy.

For example, let's say you decide to buy a car. The Emoter wants to get what it wants and feel like it is a good choice, regardless of the consequences in the future. If the Thinker is Active, it might start doing things like looking at your budget, calculating your retirement savings or checking the balance of your emergency fund. You know, horribly annoying things that involve the future.

Passive Thinker Car Buying

Emoter: Hey, look at this car! What a beauty!

Thinker: That's $5 thousand over budget.

Emoter: Whatever. It makes me feel warm and tingly inside. I gotta have it. Make it so.

Thinker: Well, looks like it is a *Consumer Reports Best Buy* and has an excellent quality rating. This car will pay for itself when we save money on all the repairs we won't have to do.

Emoter: Great point! And gosh darn it, I deserve it – it's about time I started making what I want important!

Thinker: The problem is, we don't have the money.

Emoter: Solve it man!

Thinker: I guess we could finance it.

We don't like to make choices we feel are wrong, so we find a way to have them feel right.

The Thinker Can Be Ignored, the Emoter Can't

We have an amazing ability to justify just about anything but sometimes we can't do it. In these cases, we just tune out the Thinker. We numb it, anesthetize it, drug it, distract it, or find any way we can to just not think about what our actions are going to create. If we can't find a way to convince ourselves that our behavior is okay, we have to ignore the future completely.

Look at extreme cases of self-destructive behavior. People get to six hundred pounds, spend themselves into $100 thousand worth of debt, or stay in unhealthy relationships or jobs long after they've run out of ways to justify their behaviors. They no doubt have a long list of justifications but often they don't even run through that internal mental B.S. (Basic Story) anymore. They just don't think about it at all.

Most of us can relate to times when we knew that what we were doing was wrong and just turned off our awareness of the future. This is essentially putting the Thinker to sleep. "Ah to heck with it," we say and just do what the Emoter wants. As humans, we can develop an almost unbelievable ability to live in denial and distraction, and devote large sums of time and money to finding ways to ignore what is going on in our lives.

Active Thinker Mode

Here is a classic example of Active versus Passive thinking. Cross your arms, then uncross them and cross them again in the opposite way.

Really, put the book down and try it.

Now for the few of you who actually did that, when you first crossed your arms, the Robot performed the action because it's a pattern that requires no conscious thought. In other words, the Thinker was not needed. Then, when you tried to cross them the opposite way, the Robot said, "I've got nothing." The Thinker had to step in and work it out. You have just experienced what it feels like to switch on your Thinker.

In his book, *The Power of Habit – Why We Do What We Do in Life and Business,* Charles Duhigg tells the story of a remarkable woman named Lisa Allen. She pulled off an amazing transformation of her life, going from a thirty-year-old who:

> "Had started smoking and drinking when she was sixteen, and had struggled with obesity for most of her life. At one point, in her mid-twenties, collection agencies were hounding her to recover $10,000 in debts. An old résumé listed her longest job as lasting less than a year."

Four years later:

> "A lean and vibrant woman, with the toned legs of a runner. She looked a decade younger than the photos in her chart and like she could out-exercise anyone in the room. According to the most recent report in her file, Lisa had no outstanding debts, didn't drink, and was in her thirty-ninth month at a graphic design firm."

In an interview with one of the many scientists who like to study her uncommon transformation, Duhigg writes:

> "I want to show you one of your most recent scans," a researcher told Lisa near the end of her exam. He pulled up a picture on a computer screen that showed images from inside her head. "When you see food, these areas"— he pointed to a place near the center of her brain—"which are associated with craving and hunger, are still active. Your brain still produces the urges that made you overeat. "However, there's new activity in this area"— he pointed to the region closest to her forehead [Thinker]—"where we believe behavioral inhibition and self-discipline starts. That activity has become more pronounced each time you've come in."

What Lisa had managed to do was take a behavior driven by the Robot and the Emoter and move it to the Thinker. She not only put her Thinker into Active mode, but she also had documented proof that over time, she had built a stronger and more active Thinker.

We need to understand that the Thinker has two modes: the Passive mode, when it is a servant of the Emoter, and the Active mode. In this mode, the Thinker is able to moderate urges and impulses, and to regulate emotions, basically keeping the Emoter in check. We don't do this through will-power; we do this through effective Emoter management. In other words, we don't override the Emoter, we steer it in a better direction. We learn to effectively collaborate with the Emoter rather than fight it.

Active Thinker Car Buying

Emoter: Hey, look at this car! What a beauty!

Thinker: That's $5 thousand over budget.

Emoter: Whatever. It makes me feel warm and tingly inside. I gotta have it. Make it so.

Thinker: True, warm and tingly, but so does having money to pay our bills.

Emoter: Right. Sure. Good point. Want the car.

Thinker: Let's find the same car that's a couple of years old. Let somebody else pay for the new car depreciation.

Emoter: But then it will be used! It won't smell new.

Thinker: This one will be used in a week and won't smell new in a month. How about we get one of those "new car smell" car fresheners?

Emoter: Ooo. And fuzzy dice.

Thinker: No.

Notice the Active Thinker did something very important here. It used the future to change how the Emoter feels now.

> **When in Active Thinker mode, we hold the present in one hand and the future in the other. We focus on both *now* and *later*. The problems come when we ignore either.**

You ignore later if you over-eat, over-spend or over-schedule. The immediate is the only thing that matters. You ignore now when you use will-power to force yourself to do something that you don't want to do. The trick is to keep both now and later in focus. I'll go more deeply into this in Part Three.

When in Active mode, the Thinker is working much harder than when the Robot is in charge. As such, there is a time limit for how long the Thinker can be Active. This time limit can be expanded through building a stronger Thinker, but there will always be a limit. Therefore, we have a two-part strategy. First, build a better Thinker through awareness, understanding, and use. Second, learn how to reprogram the Robot so you can change at those times when you are automatically and unconsciously producing results you don't want. More on this also in Part Three.

You want the Thinker to be in charge as much as possible and to have a Robot you can rely on to take over when it needs a rest.

> **The primary job of an ACTIVE Thinker is to be in touch with present reality, and to track the future you are creating.**

Summary

The Thinker is the analogy we will use to represent the functions of your brain that handle reasoning, problem solving, predicting the future, and critical thinking. It is the part of your brain that has the ability to override past conditioning, challenge assumptions, project a series of events into the future to predict an outcome, and collaborate with the Emoter to make the best possible decisions.

The Thinker has two modes that it operates in: Passive and Active. In Passive mode, the Thinker takes direction from the Emoter and is primarily concerned with getting the Emoter what it wants as soon as possible, without regard for future consequences. The Passive Thinker will:

- Allow the Robot to go unchecked
- "Adjust Perceptions" to help the Emoter be right
- Justify almost any action
- Be ignored completely if the previous two efforts fail

The Active Thinker will do the opposite. It will challenge the Robot's view of the world and work to get past bias and preconceived notions, thus moving beyond being "right." It will calculate the effect and future consequences of choices and work with the Emoter so that it is not ignored.

The Active Thinker holds the present in one hand and the future in the other, then finds a way to make them co-exist.

There is a time limit to how long the Thinker can be Active because it consumes more energy this way. As a result, the two-fold approach is to build a stronger Thinker to increase the amount of time spent Active, and to reprogram the Robot when ineffective patterns are found so that the Robot can be relied upon more often.

4

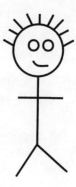

I AM the Boss of You!
The Emoter

"Let's not forget that the little emotions are the great captains of our lives and we obey them without realizing it."
- Vincent Van Gogh, 1889

In an odd marriage of seemingly disconnected fields, the 2002 Nobel Prize in economics was awarded to a psychologist named Daniel Kahneman. He was able to prove that people make decisions for emotional reasons first, and then use logic to justify their choices. This finding turned the economics field on its head because it had tons of models based on the assumption that people would make decisions that made sense. His work has spawned an entirely new field called Behavioral Economics.

A gentleman in one of my courses questioned this finding, saying, "I can see how, when I've been angry, I've said things or done things I wish I hadn't, and I can see how emotions were in charge. But when it comes to money management, I'm very rational in how I manage my finances. So, is it not always true?"

I said, "Let me ask you some questions about your money. Are you debt free? Do you have a retirement plan? Can you go six months without income?" Basic financial health questions most people can't answer. He said, yes. Then I asked him if he had a credit card. He said, "Yes, and if I use it, at the end of the month, I pay it off."

I then asked, "How would it feel to carry a balance on that card?" He said, "It would feel awful. I don't know how people live that way." So, is paying off that card a logical or emotional choice?

For him it was actually both. His emotions and his logic were in sync, so when he looked at his actions, all he saw was the logic of paying off the card and that logic covered up or disguised the emotion of how awful he would feel carrying debt. He made an emotional choice that he thought was for logical reasons. We only tend to see the emotion when we can't rationalize our actions, and as it turns out, we are very good at rationalizing just about anything.

The bottom line is the Emoter is the source of our motivations, much more so than logic. All three drivers are hugely important but we will find that the Emoter is going to be our key to success in eliminating the Never Enough Mindset.

The Will Power Myth

On occasion, frustrated by our apparent inability to get ourselves to do the things we think we should do, we knuckle down and turn on some *will power*. This is when we force ourselves into the action that the Emoter doesn't want to do. We force ourselves to go to the gym; we swear to not procrastinate anymore; we start yet another diet; we resolve to make and stick to a budget; you name it. This lasts three months, three days or for some, three minutes, and we revert back. Then we torture ourselves internally with another shame and guilt session: "You're so lazy. You have no will power!"

The truth is, will power as a method for long-term change rarely works. The reason is quite simple: going against the Emoter is a losing battle. We need to learn to work with the Emoter, not against it – not suppress, deny or control. The people who are good at what others call will power or self-discipline are actually good at managing the Emoter, rather than over-riding or getting rid of emotions. Or it could just be that their Emoter happens to enjoy the action they are taking, so for them there is no need to over-ride it or manage it in the first place.

For example, if you ask someone who exercises on a regular basis, "How do you make yourself do it? How do you manage to push through the misery of your life day after day?" They, of course, don't describe exercise as something they have to *make* their Emoter do; their Emoter *wants* to do it. It's the people whose Emoters don't enjoy exercise who figure the only way forward is to force themselves to do something they don't want to do, or find a way to bury or turn off the emotion.

If we could bury our emotions, what would our lives be like? Some people would say corporate America. It seems that the business world has been trying for many years to rid people of the nuisance of emotions while they work. "Be professional," really means, "Be emotionless." This ignoring of, or denying the necessity of the Emoter's role, has created some bleak, depressed, and joyless places to work. And even more important to a results-driven organization – ignoring or denying emotions doesn't actually get better results in the long run. It really just gets in the way of creating great results. Our aim is to guide our emotions to work for us, rather than against us.

Fear and Desire

Here's a question for you. How many colors are there? Thousands? Millions? More? Actually, there are only three: the primary colors that combine to form the huge array of different colors that we perceive. I think the same analogy can be used to understand emotions at the simplest level. While we experience a wide variety of emotions, I believe there are really just two: fear and desire. Our fears drive us to avoid or move away from what we don't want, while our desires drive us to move toward or experience what we do want. If you really want to understand what makes your Emoter tick, know that you are basically driven by your fears, desires or some combination of the two.

This is really good news. We are driven primarily by our Emoter, and our Emoter is really just motivated by two forces: fear and desire. This greatly simplifies managing the Emoter. There are two problems though: 1) we usually don't know or want to know what we're afraid of and, 2) we often don't know what we really want. Let's look at both in more detail.

Fear

"Scaredy Cat! Scaredy Cat!" Most of us were on the receiving end of this chant or something similar as kids – maybe even last week at work. This was the early programming we received regarding the rules about fear.

"You shouldn't have it. If you do have it, don't show it and for goodness' sake, don't talk about it." Yet there is not one of us who goes through a day without experiencing fear. So here we are, running around, experiencing fear on a regular basis, and pretending we don't. The result is that most people don't know when they are having a true fear response. They think it is something else.

Because we don't have permission to experience fear, and we experience it anyway, fear surfaces in other ways. It shows up as anger, negativity, jealousy, sadness, etc. Or we suppress the fear and the effect is depression, boredom, shut-down, withdrawal, etc. It can drive us to do destructive things to ourselves and others, and it can also drive us to do good things. In short, it's a big driving force behind our actions and we need to understand it. I think you will find that fear is the strongest behavioral motivator in the world. Most people are guided more by their fears than their desires.

Fear is about survival. Its function is to keep us alive. When a caveman heard a rustling in the bushes, he learned to be wary of it. If he wasn't, he was lunch. He developed a response that would give him the maximum chance of survival when a sharp pointy-toothed beast came charging out of those bushes. The fear response releases hormones into the blood stream that increases heart rate, opens blood flow to the muscles, and reduces blood flow to non-essential functions like digestion, tissue repair, and the brain – all stuff that needs blood, but not right now because if we don't get away, those things won't matter. This is why, when some people get scared, they faint. The blood needed for their brain was redirected elsewhere. If it were caveman times, they would be helping some nice lion cubs grow big and strong. Today, they just look silly giving that presentation at work.

Here we have a physiological, biological, deeply ingrained response that no longer serves the purpose it was developed for. Most of our fear responses today are to situations that do not require a fight or flight reaction but we use them anyway because the Emoter doesn't know the difference between real or imagined life-threatening situations. Fear feels like fear, no matter the cause, so when the Emoter is in charge and feeling scared, we tend to react in ways that end up getting in the way of the results we want.

Fear and the Passive Thinker

When the Thinker is Passive, fear is often the most dominant and invisible driving force in our lives. But since the Thinker is not in charge, those fears are often baseless, misleading or downright irrational. Case in point: cats. It used to be that when Fluffy got itself stuck up a tree, people would call the Fire Department to come rescue it. As Jim loves to point out though, you don't ever see cat bones hanging from the top of a tree. The cat finds a way to get itself down sooner or later.

In Passive Thinker, there is no reality check on our fears, so our fears are disconnected from what is real. This causes us to avoid risk, and to experience stress, anxiety, and tension when we are perfectly safe.

On the other side of the coin, we learn to disregard situations that should have us so terrified that we can't help but act, like being deeply in debt, horribly out of shape or insanely over-scheduled. When the Emoter is driving, it can learn to ignore some amazingly dangerous situations.

Fear and the Active Thinker

Fear is a good thing. It keeps us safe and can add value to our lives. The problem is that most of the time when we feel fear, we are not really in danger but we respond as though we are. That's because the Thinker doesn't analyze those fears when Passive, it's out of the game. When the Thinker is Active, we can analyze things like cause and effect, and probabilities.

For example, Jim and I spend a lot of time flying. This is not something we do for our Emoter because it is not fun. Flying is something we do because it helps us achieve the purpose of our careers. Someone sitting next to me once asked, "Aren't you afraid of flying?" I said, "No, I'm good at math." I pointed out that if death is what she is afraid of, she should have been more frightened driving to the airport. This didn't seem to help her.

Being in Active Thinker mode doesn't alleviate our fears but it does make them far less likely to get in the way of living the life we want to live. To the credit of the person on that plane with me, she was there, even though she was scared. She got on the plane in the first place either because her Active Thinker worked out that it was not a fear worth acknowledging, and/or her Emoter's desire for the outcome of the action was greater than the fear.

In Active Thinker, our fears work to keep us safe because the ones that affect our actions the most are legitimate dangers. While in Passive mode, we nullify things that are not worth avoiding, or that we might even need to do.

The other aspect of fear that shows up while in Active Thinker is more positive. We can actually use fear for good. When the Thinker analyzes what is really going on, we get busy on things that the Passive Thinker overlooks. When we pay attention to our real results, it becomes very difficult to avoid our physical, financial or stress health.

> **When Active, we can ignore perceived threats that are not really dangerous and pay attention to, and be motivated by, real dangers.**

Desire

Fear in the brain is pretty straightforward and easy to map. Brain scans of people having a fear response show a very active Limbic system. This is toward the base of the brain and is the same wiring that all animals have. Where desire originates in the brain is less obvious.

The first and most simple source of desire comes from the pleasure centers of the brain, basically from our senses. When something we taste, touch, smell, hear or see is beneficial, we experience pleasure. We then want more of it. This is the most basic Emoter drive: to experience sensory pleasure.

The second source of desire comes from less direct stimulation. Feelings like love, accomplishment, acceptance, etc., are not as simple as a response in the pleasure centers of the brain. Brain scans show that when someone experiences feelings of love, activity fires in multiple areas of the brain, including the frontal cortex where the Thinker lives. Emotions are more complicated desires and I've found conflicting research on what is going on in the brain, but for the most part, researchers want to boil all desire responses down to one culprit: dopamine.

The science of dopamine goes deep and wide and is beyond the scope of this book or my expertise but the simplest explanation goes something like this: when we have an experience we enjoy, whether it's physical pleasure or emotions, dopamine is released into the brain. The exact effect of this gets complicated, but in short, we like it. We then form memories that cause us to go back to that event. An animal remembers where in the forest it found water or berries, or we remember our favorite restaurant or best friend, all because they triggered the release of dopamine.

Dopamine seems to be the brain's way of getting us to remember to go back to things that were good for us. This is helpful for a squirrel but for us it can cause problems. There is a ton of current research that explores the link between dopamine and addiction. If we could control what triggers the dopamine response, we could really get a handle on the temptations and cravings we experience.

The main reason for this science digression is to help you understand that once this trigger-reward program fueled by dopamine is set in place, it is difficult to root out and change.

Once the program is in place, all it takes is a simple trigger and the Emoter is activated. It could be the time of day, a smell or just a thought, and the craving is launched. When I used to work in an office, I would feel an urge to buy a snack from the vending machine at 3pm every day. When smokers feel a spike in emotions, high or low, they crave nicotine. When some people think of the mall, they want to shop. All these triggers create a feeling of wanting and longing for the release of the dopamines that will come with the activity. Until we get that dopamine, it will be hard to ignore the craving.

What does all this mean for our purposes of eliminating the Never Enough Mindset and mastering our health, wealth, and stress? Functionally, the analogy of Thinker, Emoter, and Robot are the same. It's all going to come down to changing your Robot, so that the Emoter has a different response. Dopamine is what makes the Emoter tick at the deepest level, but it is an unconscious desire, and all we know is that we crave something. So, for the sake of simplicity, and with apologies to the scientific community, we're going to call this part the desire drive in the Emoter. In practice, this will work, even if it is an oversimplification.

Desire and the Passive Thinker

When the Emoter is calling the shots, our desires act like a three-year old saying, "I want it! I want it!" These desires are: 1) disconnected from what it will take to get them, and 2) don't take into account the consequences of getting them.

In the first assertion, people fantasize about big beautiful houses, a nicer car, a different body or a new spouse, all without considering what it would take to get those things. We dream of winning the lottery with no regard for the statistics involved. In Passive Thinker mode, what it would take to achieve the desired outcome is ignored.

The second issue we ignore is the consequence of the outcome. I want to buy something and don't consider the cost. I want to eat and don't think about what it will do to my body. Companies chase quarterly profits without considering the big picture. When Passive, the Thinker does not assess the consequences of attaining the desired outcome, so those consequences do not affect the Emoter's longing for the outcome.

Desire and the Active Thinker

When Active, the Thinker works out what it will take to achieve an outcome and what the consequence of that outcome will be. Doing so changes what the Emoter wants.

> **When the Active Thinker looks at the work of attaining something and the consequences of achieving it, our feelings change about that outcome.**

When we don't think about the cost, monthly payments or retirement, the Emoter picks a great big beautiful house we probably can't afford. The way to change the desire for that house, is to have the future effect of that choice make an impact on our emotions right now. When the Active Thinker looks at dessert, it doesn't just see yummy food, it sees larger clothes or extra work to burn it off.

Our emotional state is changed by including the future in our thinking, rather than just the present. We are still driven to go after our desires, and that's okay. But it's best to go for it with our eyes open, with an accurate picture of what it will take to get it, and a realistic appraisal of the effect of the outcome.

Summary

The Emoter is the construct we will use to represent the feelings and emotions you experience, and to illuminate their effect. The Emoter is the boss of you. Stop trying to change that and get to know your boss. That you are primarily driven by your emotions is not the problem. The problem comes from being driven ONLY by your emotions. We tend to feel first and then use lines of reasoning to justify the actions we want. You can learn to think and feel at the same time.

I'm not going to have you put the Emoter in the back seat and try to make it be quiet. You are going to learn to have the Thinker drive and have the Emoter be an active co-pilot and motivator. To succeed at this, you have to understand your fears and desires, so that you know what the Emoter is after. You can then pick better strategies for getting the Emoter what it wants without creating damage.

5

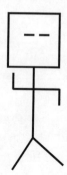

"It's Not My Fault Dad! It's a Habit!" The Robot

People are funny when they talk about habits. They see them as unstoppable forces. They'll say things like, "It's a habit, what are ya' gonna' do?" Even my son: when he was six, he learned how to talk while breathing in instead of while breathing out. It was maddening. I asked him to stop doing that, and he said, "It's not my fault DAD! It's a habit!" As if that was the end of the conversation.

Habits are seen as unmovable because they are rooted in the Robot. To change a habit, we will be reprogramming or even redesigning the Robot, changing the very foundation of our thoughts, feelings, and behaviors. We are lousy at changing habits because we are terrible at changing the Robot.

The Robot represents everything in the brain that comes from the past. What the Emoter feels and the Thinker thinks comes from a combination of what is going on right now, and what the Robot has to say about it. But the Robot is speaking from past experiences. The way we were raised, the events and experiences we've had, the environments we've been in, and the people we've been around have all affected us in some way. We have formed beliefs, opinions, values, memories, perceptions, etc. They all blend together to profoundly, and often invisibly, shape our behaviors.

New Tricks for Old Dogs

You've probably heard of the age-old nurture vs. nature debate. How much of who we are comes from what we experience over our lifetime versus what we are pre-determined to become, given our genetic makeup. For many years, the common position held by the community of human behavior scientists, was that we are a relatively blank slate at birth and our parenting, environment, and conditioning determine the behaviors we will exhibit later in life. Newer research shows that our genetic makeup plays a much bigger role than previously thought.

Identical twins separated at birth and raised in completely different families and environments, even in different parts of the world, end up having amazingly similar traits and characteristics. Ask any parent if part of personality is inborn and they will say, "Yes." In our case, my wife and I are quite certain there are aspects to our son's personality that were there long before we had a chance to mess him up.

How much of who we are is nature vs. nurture? I certainly can't say for sure. There is compelling evidence to suggest that both play a significant role, but I don't have the answer and I don't think anyone else does either. For the most part, I also think it doesn't matter. You are who you are now and need to work forward from that. What matters most is, can you change? If not, there is not much point in this book and we can't have that, so let's conclude that you *can* change. You can find a way to become who you want to be, and that will end up incorporating your unique and unchangeable genetic makeup. You will find a way to make whatever can't be changed work for you.

The great news is that the latest research shows that our minds are much more malleable than was previously thought, meaning we can change the conditioning that has shaped the Robot as well.

The Robot's Main Functions

It is estimated that eighty percent of our core beliefs are formed by age five. Obviously, we adopt many beliefs after we're five, so here is the analogy. Imagine you are going to build a house. You start by clearing the land, putting in some rough plumbing, pouring a foundation, and erecting the framing. This can all be done in less than a month, but that house won't be done for at least another two or three months, and probably more. The wiring, plumbing, sheetrock, flooring, cabinetry, contractor lawsuits, etc., all need to be done, but the original foundation and framing will determine what that house is going to look like.

By five years old, we have a basic belief system, just like a house has a framework. We already have a concept about how safe the world is; we know if we are loved; we have an idea that good things are going to happen to us. In the case of our son, once he turned six, I could start to see his thinking change from figuring out the world and being full of questions, to putting everything he learned into perspective relative to what he already knew. He went from being a curious guy to being a mister know-it-all, smarty-pants.

Even though our core Robot structures are already formed at an early age, we can change them, but the deeper they are and the more other beliefs and constructs are based on them, the harder they are to alter.

The Robot serves four main functions:

- Auto Pilot
- Alarm System
- Database Manager
- Screen Manager

Each of these functions has been in place for a long time. We don't think about them; they just happen automatically and unconsciously. We can be consciously aware of what we are thinking and feeling, but the Robot works in the background. With practice, we can get better at noticing some of what the Robot is doing, but not all of it. There is simply too much going on. The good news is that we don't have to know everything. We are only concerned with the behaviors the Robot does that are not working for us. We really just need to isolate the faulty or outdated programming and correct it. Understanding each of the main functions of the Robot and how they work will make it easier for us to identify where the bugs exist in the code.

Auto Pilot

How much of your day is run by the Robot? It can be hard to say because when the Robot is in charge, we are, by definition, not thinking about it. As mentioned before, one study put it at forty percent, but I think it is usually more. This is the part of the Robot people are most familiar with but also have the hardest time identifying. We know we do things by habit, unconsciously, but how do those behaviors get there, and how do we spot them and change them if we have a hard time seeing them?

There was a movie in the nineteen-eighties called *War Games*. The opening scene of the movie showed two guys sitting in a bunker under a nuclear missile silo. All the silos used to have this setup and the guys would basically sit there and wait for the order to come in to fire their missiles. The sirens started going off and the guys began their practiced routine to fire, running through their checklist and verifications and so on. Both guys had a key, and in order to launch their rocket, they both had to insert their keys and turn them at the same time on different sides of the room. This way, one guy couldn't just freak out and decide to fire away. In the movie, when the time comes to turn their keys, one guy does and the other doesn't. He decides he just can't bring himself to do it. The other guy is pointing a gun at him, screaming, "Turn your key!" But he refuses. The sirens stop. It was just a drill and that guy probably got fired.

This becomes a great analogy for how the Robot decides to store information because, just like the missile, both keys in your head have to be turned before the Robot will change. In your head though, the two that hold the keys are the Thinker and the Emoter.

The story in your head might go something like this:

Thinker: We need to exercise. Let's go to the gym.

Emoter: We've been over this. Exercise bad. Do your thing so I don't have to.

(Thinker clubs the Emoter over the head, stuffs it into a bag, and puts it in the trunk, then gets in the car and starts driving to the gym. In other words, it uses will-power.)

Thinker: Robot, remember this behavior. We are going to exercise three times a week.

Robot: Okay. Key turn detected. Waiting for additional input.

(Emoter says from the trunk.)

Emoter: I'm not turning my key! No way! Get me out of here! I'm not going to no stupid gym!

(Three weeks later, the Thinker gives up.)

We will go much deeper into changing the Robot in Chapter 8, but for now, the biggest reason most people struggle to create lasting change is that they don't find a way for the Emoter to turn its key. It becomes a Thinker-only behavior, which is will power, and after the Thinker runs out of steam, the behavior reverts back to the original, unmodified pattern in the Robot. It returns to what is familiar. This is the main point to understand about the auto pilot function of the Robot:

> ## The Robot will not take in new programming unless both the Thinker AND Emoter agree.

Why does the Auto Pilot function of the Robot even exist? One word: efficiency. A behavior driven by the Robot consumes considerably less energy than when the Thinker has to do it. For example, I travel a lot. One day, we were going on vacation so my wife and son were traveling with me. At one point during the process of getting to our gate, my wife said, "You don't really like traveling with us, do you?" I, of course, thought, "What a horrible thing to say." But sadly, she was right. I love going on vacation with my family, but the traveling part, not so much.

The reason is that my Robot can get me from my couch, to the airport, and through connections. It can pick up a rental car, find my hotel, and get me up and ready to present the next day, all without the use of my Thinker. I read my Kindle standing in the security line. I have the layout of most airports I go through memorized. I don't like traveling, so when I have my pattern disturbed, like getting my wife and her three different bottles of liquid that she forgot she had in her carry-on, through security, my Robot leaves Auto Pilot mode and fires off an alarm; my Emoter gets grumpy and my Thinker has to take over.

This energy-saving feature is very useful, because having to consciously think our way through every action of every day would be exhausting. The down side comes when patterns and programs get put into the Robot that don't produce the results we want. The Robot doesn't think, it just carries out the pattern, regardless of the outcome.

The Robot's Auto Pilot gets triggered by certain events or situations. For example, 3pm used to trigger me to go to the vending machine at work and get some M&M's. Smokers get triggered to have a cigarette when they feel a spike in emotion, like stress or even happiness. Something as simple as boredom can trigger an urge to eat or drink. When you begin changing your ways, you're going to have to reprogram your Auto Pilot.

Alarm System

This is the warning function of The Robot. The sirens will go off when the Robot senses something it perceives to be a danger, such as an unexpected loud noise, or engaging in an activity that is unfamiliar. Our comfort zones determine when the Alarm System goes off, making it difficult to leave those familiar zones and create new results. Our Alarm System keeps us safe but it also keeps us from changing.

For example, remember a time when someone startled you. What did you do? You jumped, twitched, yelled, and maybe smacked them. None of these behaviors had anything to do with The Thinker or The Emoter, although they were probably pretty active afterwards. The Robot sounded the alarm because it sensed danger, which is probably okay in this situation. But it will also sound the alarm when it faces a new challenge, which can cause problems.

When faced with a new situation or challenge, the Robot sounds an alarm because it doesn't have a pattern that it can plug in and follow. Even if that behavior is something you want to do, the Robot still sounds the alarm. The Robot is simply saying that it doesn't know how to respond in this situation. When faced with the unknown, we tend to go to a fear response. We can respond to it with our Emoter, which will go down the fight or flight road, or we can respond with the Thinker. We tend to use the Emoter, and the net effect of the alarm signal is to move us away from the new situation, and back into the familiar.

Some examples of this: most people who lose weight on a diet gain it back, and then some. Over seventy percent of lottery winners go bankrupt, and most people who do debt consolidation end up deeper in debt. These are examples of people who moved out of their comfort zones and then found a way back in.

> ## It is easier to return to familiar patterns than it is to learn new ways.

The alarm response is a good thing because it helps keep us safe. At times though, the Robot sounds false alarms, going off when we are not really in danger. We need to learn to identify when the Robot is doing this and develop better strategies for responding to it. In other words, we need to learn how to operate outside our comfort zones. Only by experiencing the new, unknown, and unfamiliar can we create effective change. More on how to do this in Chapter 8.

Database Manager

Another important feature of our Robot is memory. The Robot is our own dictionary and encyclopedia. For the younger crowd that doesn't know what one of those is, look it up on Wikipedia, which is an even better analogy for the Robot because, just like what's in the Robot, the information isn't necessarily true. Unfortunately, the Robot often records things inaccurately.

Memory itself is a very large topic with entire books and even university departments devoted to the subject. There is, however, one main concept related to memory that is most relevant to this offering, which is, we are not so good at remembering things.

From Science Daily (Sep. 20, 2000):

"In one experiment, the researchers showed a short clip from a contemporary film to 53 people (45 percent men, 55 percent women). The clip involved a married couple arguing over the husband's extramarital affair while their young daughter looks on. About half of the research participants were instructed to watch the clip and not let their feelings show as they watched (expressive suppression group). Participants in the control group were instructed only to watch and listen carefully to the clip.

Results showed that even though the two groups showed no difference in their emotional experience, participants in the expressive suppression group had poorer memory for what was said and done in the clip than did the control participants."

The group that was suppressing their Emoters remembered less. Where were you on 9/11? Almost everyone can answer. Quick, where were you on 9/5? Unless that was a big day for your Emoter as well, you don't remember it. You can think of emotions as the glue that holds memories in place. People don't remember what you told them, they remember how you made them feel. What really happens is that the Emoter dictates to the Robot, and the only facts that are stored are the ones needed to frame and explain the emotions that were felt.

The stronger the Emoter's response, the more we remember.

I could give many more examples but I'll save you the trouble and share what my research has found. The Emoter messes up our ability to remember stuff correctly. Because of this, we need to be dubious of our memories and know that they are distorted for a wide variety of reasons. This is a problem because, as we will see in the next section, we rely on our Robot's Database quite heavily.

Screen Manager

Most people go through life believing that the emotions they experience are based on the events going on around them; in fact, this is not the case.

The information we receive from the world comes through our senses: taste, touch, smell, sight, and sound. We are constantly bombarded with massive amounts of data that flows to us through these senses. This is an overwhelming amount of information that, if we had to process it on a moment-to-moment basis, would consume all our attention. Fortunately, we don't have to. The information from our senses does not go to the Emoter or the Thinker, it goes to the Robot. The Robot takes all the information and uses stored memories and beliefs (our database) to decide what information to ignore, what information to pass along and, most importantly, what that information means.

Having sorted through the sensory data and selected what is worth paying attention to right now, the Robot projects an image on a "screen" that the Emoter looks at. This image is not a true picture of what is going on; it is an edited, colored, and distorted interpretation. The image that the Emoter is actually reacting to has had meaning assigned to it, based on the Robot's often distorted memory of past experiences. If you were to take one, and only one thing from this book, I would want it to be an understanding of how your screen works.

For example, let's say that every time you came across a person wearing a purple T-shirt, they punched you in the nose. I'm not saying this has happened, but if it did, and right now a person walked up to you wearing a purple T-shirt, what would your reaction be? Run screaming, duck and cover, call for your mom, whatever. Would this reaction be based on what is currently happening in front of you? No. The Emoter's response would be based on what it saw on the screen, and that would be a picture of it getting punched in the nose.

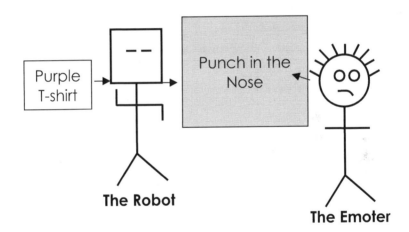

This example might be a little silly, but now consider what image your Robot puts on the screen when you consider money, food, your boss, marriage, etc. In the quest for emotional mastery, you must understand that the emotions you experience are not directly connected to the events going on around you; your emotions are a reaction to the image presented to you by the Robot.

This image has also been referred to as our context, paradigm, perspective or point of view. For many though, this image is treated as *THE TRUTH*, when in fact, it is our narrow slice of the truth of the moment, distorted and influenced by our past.

This distortion spins the picture one way or another. Sometimes the spin makes the image look better than things really are; sometime the spin makes things look worse. Either way, to create change in your life, you're going to have to become more conscious of the difference between what you are reacting to and the reality before you.

Some more examples of how this screen works:

Let's say you get some positive feedback but you tend to have a hard time accepting compliments. Your Boss says, "Hey, great job on that project last week. You're really a rising star." The Emoter doesn't react to this. What the Emoter reacts to is the Robot's interpretation of what was said.

Robot: Our Boss said the project last week was not horrible, and it looks like he wants something. I have given automated response, "Thank you. I really appreciate that."

Emoter: Oh boy. I wonder what he wants now. I bet I'm in trouble.

Now let's say you get some critical feedback and tend to be less than compassionate with yourself. Your Boss says, "Looks like there was a mistake on the report you turned in yesterday. Page two, the numbers are reversed on the graph. Otherwise, looks pretty good."

Robot: Our Boss says we did a really horrible job on the report.

Emoter: Oh no! Thinker, come up with something good to say!

Thinker: "My bad. I'll fix it and get it back to you later today."

Emoter: Great! There goes our raise. He probably wants to fire me now. Ah, I'm such an idiot!

Now consider an example of what happens when two screens collide. Jim was driving down the road one day when someone cut him off.

Robot: The car in front of us turned sharply into our lane. The Database suggests that he hates us and wants us to die.

Emoter: Scream things at him and make gestures! (Response edited for appropriateness.)

(Jim's wife, Brenda is in the car with him. She says, "I'll bet he's rushing to the hospital to be with his sick child.")

Robot: Wife unit is offering a different interpretation of the event.

Emoter: Does it match ours precisely?

Robot: No, not at all.

Now at this point, Jim had some different roads he could have chosen. He could have just given up, which might have looked like this:

Emoter: Well that guy is a jerk, no question. Can't say that. Thinker, get to work.

Thinker: "I hadn't considered that honey. Good thought."

He could have carefully considered why their Robots had such different interpretations and had a meaningful discussion about that. Or he could have gone with the most common approach that most people use when their Robot's view of the world is challenged, and argued that he was right, which is what he did. He said something like, "No way. That guy is a jerk." To which Brenda replied, "What makes your fantasy any more real than mine?"

Different Robots putting up different images on screens are the cause of much confusion and conflict in the world.

The Screen Management role of the Robot is a double-edged sword. It is very effective at sifting through a mountain of data in real-time, almost instantaneously, then deciding what information to notice and pass along to the Thinker and the Emoter. The down side is that sometimes the Robot will ignore information that would help us or that we may need; at other times it will warp or twist the data at hand. This is where bias and prejudice come from.

The main criteria the Robot uses when filtering information is, does it match? The Robot tends to analyze what it perceives, pass along information that matches the existing beliefs and memories stored in the database, and reject the rest. So, to change habits, the Thinker is going to have to learn how and when to override the Robot to allow in new information that might be needed. We will expand on this in Chapter 7, Rule #2 – Be Right About the Right Things.

Summary

The Robot is the analogy we will use to represent the pre-programmed and unconscious functions of our brain. Your Robot is an amazing and important character in your Internal Game. Without it, you would be completely overwhelmed trying to make sense of the world. Just look into the eyes of a baby; everything is a wonder. You can see the blank slate that is their Robot. Your Robot is anything but blank.

Your Robot sounds alarms that keep you safe but also keep you from growing. It performs a whole host of menial and repetitive tasks on Auto Pilot, records and stores events prioritized by the emotional weight into a database, filters out tons of information, and assigns meaning to events that give rise to your emotions and actions.

We tend to be unconscious about how our Robots get programmed, and even more unaware of how they operate. By gaining a better understanding and mastery of this machinery that continuously operates in the background, you can learn how to plant custom-designed behaviors into it that will automatically create the results you are after.

Part Two

The External Game

6

Why Too Much is Never Enough

To review from Chapter 2:

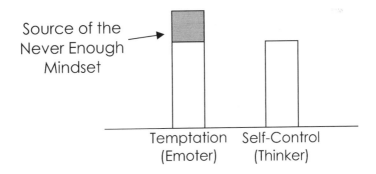

Source of the Never Enough Mindset →

Temptation (Emoter)   Self-Control (Thinker)

The Never Enough Mindset comes from the temptations we experience that exceed our current level of self-control. I've also said that this in *not* because we have gone through a kind of biological degradation that has made us a nation of simple, weak-minded people who can't control themselves like their ancestors did. We live in a very different culture and society than any that has come before us.

In this chapter, we will examine some of the factors that have unintentionally conspired to create the Never Enough Mindset. The truth is, your Emoter is under nearly constant attack; your Robot has been conditioned and programmed to perceive your life as lacking, no matter what you achieve; and your Thinker has received less growth and strengthening than those of our ancestors.

Understanding the environmental variables and influences going on around you in the External Game will help you to better master the Internal Game, and the results that flow from it.

The Declining Role of the Future

Long ago we were a nation of farmers. In fact, for almost all of modern history, we have been a species of farmers. In 1940 it took one farmer to feed about eighteen people. Today, one farmer in the U.S. feeds about one hundred and fifty-five people. That means there are a whole lot of people who have had to find a different career. We are not a nation of farmers anymore, but you can still see the remnants of it. Our school calendar for example, is still based on the farming schedule.

Where am I going with this? Farmers are good at future planning. They have to constantly think ahead. Get the fields ready, plant the crops, get ready for the harvest, harvest, prepare the fields for next year, and always have enough to get through a whole year in case the entire crop fails.

We've gone from a society that constantly thought about and planned for the future to one that thinks much more short term. It's not only the change in farming that has caused this; societal engineering programs like unemployment, social security, Medicare, and welfare have lessened the need for future planning as well. I'm not saying these are bad programs. I'm in favor of them, or at least their intention. But an unintended side effect from the societal point of view is that the average person does not *have* to be as good at thinking ahead.

The Thinker is the part of your brain that plans for the future. It is the only part of your brain that can. So, if you spend fewer of your days paying attention to the future than someone else, it stands to reason that they will have a stronger Thinker than you. The net effect is that the average person has a weaker Thinker today than in days gone by.

Most of the focus of this book is on the temptation side of the Never Enough Mindset imbalance, but remember that the other side matters as well. The approach to fixing the Never Enough Mindset is to decrease your temptations AND increase your self-control. You will learn more about building a stronger Thinker in Chapter 8.

I focus more on the temptation side because that is where most of the change has taken place. In other words, as a society our Thinkers are weaker, meaning we have less self-control; but the increase in temptations is where the major part of the problem comes from.

Marketing

Marketing is one of the biggest contributors to the temptations we experience. Marketers have become masters at finding us everywhere, then blasting us with messages that say, "Your life is not enough. Fortunately, we have the answer."

Total advertising dollars spent in 1960 was about $12 billion per year, now it's over $238 billion. In 1965, we were exposed to roughly five hundred and sixty advertisements per day. Today it's nearly three thousand.

Those marketers are good; man they are good. They know how to reach your Emoter. Ideally, your Internal Game would be so strong and solid that you would not be influenced by all these messages. In reality, very few people are skilled enough to resist this onslaught of messages. Most people are taken in, at least a little and sometimes a lot.

> ## Marketing is the art of Emoter seduction.

The good news is that you are already better prepared to handle the onslaught. Your assignment is to have your Thinker watch closely how it's done. Pay attention to the way advertising is designed and implemented to tug at your Emoter. When you can see more clearly what's going on and how it's happening, it lessens the effect. Your Emoter goes from being tempted to being annoyed and offended. "How dare they try and sucker me like that!" is the response I want you to feel.

Lead Us Into Temptation

Let's take a look at some of the temptations, other than marketing, that once didn't exist. We'll start with money. We get tons of credit card offers, home refinancing deals, payday loans, etc. We have access to debt like no nation in history. Combine that access with the demands and pressures to spend and it is no surprise that we overdo it. This level of temptation to spend combined with the ability to do so is unprecedented in human history.

The older generations like to talk about how kids today have no discipline, no will power. You know, like they did when they were young. What they don't consider though, is that in the nineteen-sixties you couldn't buy more than you could afford. If you didn't have the money, nobody was going to give you the merchandise. That's not a problem today. Back in the nineteen-sixties it wasn't as much about great internal fiscal discipline as it was about not having nearly the availability of credit we have today combined with the constant marketing and social pressure to buy. While they may have had more self-control from stronger Thinkers, they had differently programmed Robots and significantly less temptation pulling on their Emoters.

How about food? Our bodies are wired to crave salt, sugar, and fat, and the supply and demand-based free market has made those things available at a cost and density never seen before. For example, compare an apple to a Snickers bar. The Snickers bar (annual gross sales of $2 billion) weighs 57 grams, has 280 calories, 140 mg of salt, 28.8 g of sugar, and 13.6 g of fat. The apple weighs 150 grams, has 53 calories, 10.6 g of sugar, and almost no salt or fat. The extra weight is water, fiber, and nutrients that the Snickers bar does not have. Look at how much salt, sugar, and fat is packed into something nearly one-third the weight.

No doubt there are better examples and the more food savvy readers are pounding the book against a table right now (stop if you have an E-reader), but you get the point. Our food has a lesser density of the things we need like vitamins and nutrients and a greater density of the things we crave, making it much more tempting.

Today there are over 160 thousand fast food places in the United States. Fast food chains began to take off in the nineteen-sixties, so the total number of restaurants back then is skewed, but in nineteen-sixty there were only 200 McDonalds while today there are 12,804 just in the United States. The temptation for quick, cheap, less healthy food has never been higher. Our food supply is basically Emoter Crack.

One more temptation increase is the number of distractions and entertainments we are bombarded with. People used to sit on the front porch, watch the kids play, and talk to each other. Why? There was nothing else to do. The poor folks didn't know how miserable they were. Fortunately, TV came along and solved that problem. People's schedules feel crazy busy today because we have some kind of entertainment or distraction available to fill every waking minute, and lots of pressure to do so. The runaway stress most Americans experience comes in part from the never-ending list of activities we want, and that we feel obliged to put on our schedules.

We soak in a daily bath of temptation until our fingers and wallets are, as my son would say, "pruney." The better looking and more necessary it seems, the more we start to believe it will make us happier, so we lunge for it. Because some of these things are easier to get than ever before, we get them! But if there is more to have, the temptations keep getting triggered, and it just never seems to feel like enough.

Over-weight, over-spent, and over-stressed are the big three areas that are most representative of our Never Enough mentality. You can see that in each of these areas the amount of temptation you are exposed to on a daily and even hourly basis has never been greater. You will have to either reduce the amount of temptation around you, or increase your ability to manage yourself around the temptations. This book is about the latter because I don't see the amount of temptations decreasing anytime soon.

Decisions, Decisions . . .

Barry Schwartz PhD is a Swarthmore College psychologist and author of *The Paradox of Choice: Why More is*

Less. According to him, having too many choices is a bad thing. How can this be? The more choices I have, the more likely it is I'll get what I want and like what I get. This turns out not to be the case.

When you go shopping today for just about anything, how many options are there? How many different cars, TV's, houses, or even simple things like types of cereal, salad dressing, or TV channels? The belief held by most of us is that the more we have to choose from, the better. With all these choices, certainly we will be able to find a choice with which we will be happy.

One of Jim's friends from Uzbekistan once visited him. He took her to the grocery store; after five minutes she became overwhelmed and had to leave. Outside she said, "Why would anyone need twenty different kinds of peanut butter?" Jim said, "Americans like choices." She didn't understand.

The effect of many choices can lead to being unhappy with whatever we pick. The reason? We tend to compare what we chose with what we could have chosen. When we only have one choice, it will have to be enough. With a multitude of choices, we tend to think there was a better one.

Look at how much time we spend surfing TV channels. We don't know what is on the other channels so we tend to look, and with so many channels available, there is always something else that MUST be better than what we're currently watching. Sometimes we spend more time surfing than watching simply because we don't want to "miss out" on a better program.

One other problem created by all these choices, according to Dr. Schwartz is, "When you have only one choice and you are unhappy, the blame is with the world. When you have a hundred choices and you are unhappy, the fault lies with you." Our feeling of not having made the right choice erodes our belief in our ability to get what we want.

In short, the more choices you have, the more you feel like you are losing. The endless choices we have in our society are one of the forces driving the Never Enough Mindset. I think that having all these choices is a good thing; you just need to learn how to live healthily with all this abundance.

When you keep your Thinker active while making your decisions, you can manage your Emoter's response to the abundance around you and actually feel like you made the right choice. When the Emoter makes the choice with the help of a Passive Thinker, it will keep comparing what you have to the fantasy of what could have been.

Let's Go To Denmark

Year after year, the countries in Scandinavia land in the top ten on a bounty of lists about the happiest countries in the world. The people of Denmark consistently rank high on these lists, where more than two-thirds of Danes report being "very satisfied with their lives." This, according to the Eurobarometer Survey, is a figure that has held steady for more than thirty years. In studies like this, America usually lands somewhere in the top thirty or forty of the countries studied.

Other studies use a more scientific approach. Researchers at the Legatum Institute, a London-based nonpartisan think tank, set out to rank the happiest countries in the world. But because "happy" carries too much of a touchy-feely connotation, they call it "prosperity." In 2010, Legatum completed its "Prosperity Index", which ranks one hundred and ten countries, covering ninety percent of the world's population. To build its index, Legatum gathers data from twelve sources like the Gallup polling group, the Heritage Foundation, and the World Economic Forum. Each country is ranked on eighty-nine variables sorted into eight subsections: economy, entrepreneurship, governance, education, health, safety, personal freedom, and social capital. On the 2012 list, Norway is number one, Denmark is number two, and the U.S. makes it all the way up to number twelve.

Why are the Danes so much happier than Americans? Because their Robots have a built-in lower level of expectations. Americans simply expect more. Expectations and temptation are very similar. You're not as tempted by something you don't expect to get, and if you get less than you expected, you feel that you didn't get enough, just like when you have an unfulfilled temptation. The Danes' lower expectations lead to a lower level of temptation.

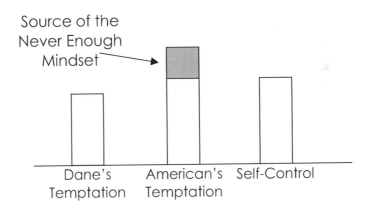

Because the Danes have low expectations, "year after year they are pleasantly surprised to find out that not everything is rotten in the state of Denmark," says James W. Vaupel, a demographer who has investigated Danish bliss.

Bliss was also a compelling topic for author Eric Weiner, who wrote *"The Geography of Bliss: One Grump's Search for the Happiest Places in the World."* Here's his take on the Danes:

> "Danes seem to know instinctively that expectations kill happiness, leaving the rest of us unhappy un-Danes to sweat it out on the "hedonic treadmill." That's what researchers call the tendency to constantly ratchet up our expectations; a sort of emotional inflation that devalues today's accomplishments and robs us of all but the most fleeting contentment. If a B-plus grade made us happy last semester, it'll take an A-minus to register the same satisfaction this semester, and so on until eventually, inevitably, we fail to reach the next bar and slip into despair."

In other words, if whatever you receive in life is at or below what you expected, it doesn't charge the Emoter. The Danes keep their expectations from increasing, so they can still satisfy their Emoters, while the expectations most Americans feel keep creeping up and up. The Danes feel like they have more than they expect to have, so they are happier. Weiner offers this quote:

Happiness = Reality - Expectations

Jim's daughter, Katelyn spent some time studying abroad in Denmark when she was in college. She was surprised to learn that in the books and movies produced in Scandinavia, very few have happy endings. Instead, they write more realistic portrayals of life. Not miserable, just accurate. The Danes compare those characters to their own lives and feel they have enough. In American movies, most characters are heroic and accuracy is hard to come by. When we compare ourselves to those characters, we don't measure up. The net, unconscious effect, is a ratcheting up of expectations.

So if the Danes are so good at expecting the life they have, does that mean they don't work to get ahead? Quite the contrary. According to the same study by the Legatum Institute, they top the list in upward mobility. The U.S. was number twelve again.

> **If you enjoy the life you have and feel like you have enough, you will still be motivated to achieve.**

America does not have a culture that lets go of expectations and that finds happiness with what is. The American mindset seems to believe that the answer lies in "more." We not only want more, we expect it. While a drive to learn, improve, and make a better life is a good thing, in order to achieve it, you don't have to be driven by a feeling that what you have is not enough.

This is a fact that many organizations don't understand. They feel that if people don't want more, they won't work hard. They attempt to dangle "more" in front of people, and then wonder why there is a lack of job satisfaction. Many companies unwittingly create Never Enough workplaces.

Another way to look at the lesson we can learn from the Danes is that they tend to live their lives with high hopes and low expectations. Americans live with higher hopes and huge expectations. Let's look at why Americans have such different hopes and expectations than the Danes.

The American Dream

What is the American Dream? I think most people would agree that the American Dream is about opportunity. In this land of opportunity, anyone can get ahead. Anyone can make a better life for themselves and their loved ones. It's a good dream, and I think it is still alive. This social experiment called America is still working pretty well when compared to any other system of government in history.

However, I believe there are two problematic side effects of the American Dream. First, as we have become a more and more prosperous nation, the list of things people hope for has grown. So the "dream" in the American Dream has steadily increased from generation to generation. We have experienced a "Dream Creep" if you will. This dream creep is where the higher hopes come from.

Dream Creep

Hundreds of years ago, what Americans dreamed of was very different. There was no electricity and there were no cars. Take those two factors away and look at the number of items on the standard American's concept of the "dream" that disappear. No TV, gaming system, computer, cell phone, second car, third car, boat, microwave, bigger refrigerator, refrigerator for the garage or basement, finished basement, pool, etc. How did they get through their days without all this stuff? Their dream was about being free from oppression, and being able to feed the family and be safe – pretty low hopes compared to today.

The other day, my family and I were taking a nighttime tour of one of those olde time villages. It was the holiday season; the paths were lit by candlelight. Christmas carolers sang and in each of the buildings were people dressed in period costumes, telling stories of what it was like to live back in those days. It was a very well done and authentic portrayal of life in the eighteen-hundreds.

I said to my ten-year-old son, Aiden, "Wow buddy. Imagine what it would be like to live like this." The houses seemed very small, and they didn't even have cable! He said to me, "Yeah, but this is all they ever had. They didn't know what life would be like with more, so they didn't feel like they were missing anything." I was a very proud father and I was left wondering, once we have more, can we ever live without it?

Early in American history, there were already signs that what people hoped for was growing. As the Royal Governor of Virginia, Lord Dunmore, noted in 1774 (*Origins of the American Revolution*, 1944), the Americans "forever imagine the Lands further off are still better than those upon which they are already settled." He added that if they attained Paradise, they would move on if they heard of a better place farther west. Already there was a dream creep going on. People were starting to want more than they had.

After World War Two, the American Dream was about getting into the middle class, and many did. People compared what they had to what the "Joneses" had. But there wasn't much difference because people compared themselves to their neighbors and other people in their own social class. If they lived in the same neighborhood, they probably had about the same income, so keeping up was doable. By comparison, people felt like they had enough. But the pressure and challenge to keep up was growing. People reached for more, hoped for more, and in many cases got it, but those hopes and dreams were creeping ever upward.

Who do we compare ourselves to today? Who have the Joneses become? They are no longer just our neighbors; now they are characters on TV, movie stars, star athletes, the latest American Idol winner or yet another reality TV personality. We've gone from dreaming of better farmland to hoping for a private jet. There was a time when almost everyone could get better farmland; not many are going to get a jet.

You might be saying, "I don't really think I'm going to get a jet." But what do you dream of? A faster computer? A new car? A bigger house? When we are exposed to so much more, it has to affect what we want for ourselves. Then if we don't get it, we feel like we don't have enough, even when we know that we do, and the Never Enough Mindset grows.

Many years ago, Jim visited Uzbekistan. People asked him about his family and he showed them a picture. They asked where he lived and he described his house. They said, "Tell us about the other people." He said, "There are only my wife and daughter." They said, "Yes, but what about the other people?" This went back and forth a few times, and finally they understood: three people lived in a five-bedroom house while they crammed three families into a one-bedroom apartment. Jim thought they must think it quite wonderful that he had such abundance. But they looked confused for a moment and then said, "That is so sad. You must be so lonely." What is enough for us is very different from most of the world.

I think there are two reasons for the dream creep. The first is that we are victims of the success of those who came before us. The more they acquired in the past, the more we think we should get today.

> ## A dream for one generation becomes an expectation for the next.

The second reason is that we are exposed to more than we used to be. People used to be aware of others who had more, but only as a concept. They rarely got a glimpse into what their lives were like. Today, we feel so familiar with people who we perceive as having more than us that we start to feel they are just like us. We don't see ourselves as peasants looking at Royalty, we see Royalty as peers. We believe we could be just like them someday, or even that we should be. "They are living the dream; why can't I?"

> ## Our picture of what we are supposed to have has vastly changed.

Expectation Creep

Earlier, I mentioned a second problem with the American Dream, and that is expectations. As we saw with the Danes, temptations increase with expectations, and our expectations have grown and grown.

> ## Buried in the American Dream is a promise for opportunity, but it can easily become an expectation.

We can get to the point where we don't just hope for our dreams but we also expect them. For example, there was a time when home ownership was a dream. Now, people feel that if they don't own a home, they are failing. Students coming right out of school want and even expect to buy a house. The reality is that some of them will move back in with their parents. It's hard to feel like that is enough if you were expecting your own house.

A little while back, I watched the President give a speech and afterwards, as is the custom, a spokesperson for the other party talked. What the spokesman said was, "The President sees us as a country of haves and have-nots. We see us as a country of haves and soon-to-haves." I thought this was a great example of what the American Dream has become because the spokesperson's message said, "You are going to have more." It's not a hope for opportunity, it's an expectation.

As the dream has soared, the pressures and expectations to achieve the dream have increased with it. The American Dream was originally a source of hope and optimism. Now, it is often an unconscious source of failure. To quote Jim on the subject, "We take a stick, paint the American dream on it, and then beat ourselves up with it."

Having big dreams isn't a problem in itself. It's when we combine huge, unrealistic dreams with expectations that they turn into nightmares.

> **We don't compare our lives to ones that are worse than our own and feel better; we compare them to ones that are better and feel worse.**

The people we hold up as winners of the American Dream are those with the most. We don't admire the achievement, we worship the having. Since we don't have as much, we end up feeling like we don't have enough.

I want to be clear that the belief that you can improve your life is a good one and is still part of the foundation that makes this a great country. Also, people have always compared themselves to others who have more or different things, so that's not new. The problem is that the difference between what we have and what we *expect* to have has increased. This creates a feeling of not having enough. The American Dream was originally about realistic hopes and low expectations, like the Danes. Somewhere along the way, it has turned into huge hopes and higher expectations.

You'll find that connecting your dreams to what can realistically happen will actually bring you fulfillment; at the same time, becoming aware of and managing your expectations, is going to be incredibly helpful in bringing your temptations under control. More on how to do that in Chapter 8.

Summary

As Americans, our Robots have been conditioned to believe that we must have more, that we deserve to have more, and that more will make us happier. Unfortunately, even when the more shows up, the happier part often does not. The net effect is the Never Enough Mindset.

If my belief is "happy lies in more," no matter what I actually get, it won't be enough. Even though we constantly pursue more, we'll never achieve happiness. We end up like a cat chasing the dot from a laser light pointer. We pounce on it, and then the next thing we know, it's over there.

What's the answer? I don't think the way to fix the problem is with external control. Strict rules on marketing, limiting our choices, controlling the food available, etc., are not approaches that I think work in most cases. The problem is not this amazing society created by those who came before us. The problem is that we don't know how to live in it in a healthy way.

I don't think will power is the answer either. Will power is about forcing ourselves to not want what we want. Maybe there are some monks sitting around in a cave somewhere who have found a way to give up wanting, but I don't want to live in a cave. My wife won't have it.

You can learn to live more happily in the world you currently have. You can learn how to be motivated by something other than *more*. You can learn to reshape your thinking so that what tempts you is within your control. This book aims to help you do that by showing you how to change at a deep level and how to experience *enough*.

7

The Rules of the Game

Games have rules, which is sometimes inconvenient. Those rules are designed for fair play, but playing by the rules doesn't necessarily make it easier to win. In sports and business, we sometimes see teams or organizations trying to skirt the rules to give themselves an advantage.

We've gone over the Internal Game and looked at the External Game; now we're going to offer some rules to follow when these two games collide. You don't have to follow the rules. No referee or government agent will knock on your door if you don't, but if you break the rules, you will definitely get into trouble – self-created trouble. Working around the rules does not give you an edge. The way to get an edge in this game is to play by the rules.

Rule #1 – Embrace Present Reality

"Agreeable as it is to know where one is proceeding, it is far more important to know where one has arrived." - John Kenneth Galbraith, The New Industrial State, 1967

In sports there is an expression: "the score doesn't lie." When the game is over, the score is the score no matter how you feel about it. I've played or watched a ton of sports during my life and many times I've seen a player complain about a call the referee or official made, yet I've never heard an official say, "Oh, you don't agree? Well I'll change the call then." The player is not putting their energy into dealing with what *is,* they are putting their energy into how *unfair* what is, is. They're not embracing present reality, they're holding onto what they think reality should be.

Someone once asked Jim, "What's the most important part of taking a trip?" Jim replied, "I think you've got to know where you're going, that's real important." The person said, "Nope, you're wrong. You need to know where you're at. If you don't know where you're at, you're lost." Or, as the Zen quote goes, "You can't get there from not here."

The most important part of any process, whether it is a trip, creating a better relationship, finding more satisfaction in your career or living a fulfilling life, is to do an honest assessment of present reality. We need that foundation of reality because any strategy built on fantasy will fail.

Guilt is one of the most common yet difficult to understand examples of how we live in denial of the present truth of our lives. Let's say I need a new pen. I go to the store, find the pen I want, go to the counter to pay for it, and discover a long line. I don't really want to wait in line, so I put the pen in my pocket and leave. When I get home, I notice the pen and feel guilty. Why would I feel guilty? Because my image of myself is that I'm not the kind of person who would steal a pen – even with the evidence staring me in the face. How would a real thief feel? "This is a great pen. Should have got a case!" But because I'm not a *real* thief, I feel guilty. As long as I can maintain my image of not being a thief while stealing, I can continue stealing without guilt. The main benefit of guilt is I don't have to look at my present reality.

The challenge in life is to put that false image of myself aside and look at my present results. So, if I have the pen that I didn't pay for, the reality is, I am a thief. As soon as I embrace present reality, I am forced to challenge my present desired reality. I'm forced to make a choice. I need to ask myself, "Do I want to be a thief?"

Jim once asked one of his groups for examples of things people feel guilty about. One man raised his hand and said that he felt guilty because he worked all the time and spent little time with his two young sons. Jim said, "So basically, on a very regular basis, you make your work more important that your sons." He got very angry and said, "They are the most important thing in my life." Jim said, "Let's look at present reality." Then he asked the man when was the last time he had something important scheduled with his sons and cancelled it for work. He said he did it all the time. Jim asked him when he last changed something he had scheduled at work to do something with his sons. He said he'd never done that and sat down. When he looked at the truth he realized that it was easier to disappoint his sons than to learn to say no to his boss.

We set strategies all the time based in fantasy. We design diet and exercise plans for someone who likes vegetables and exercise, and then we feel guilty when we eat junk food and don't exercise. We design schedules that even a workaholic couldn't master and set budgets for frugal people. What works is to embrace your reality – whatever that is. Design a diet and exercise program for someone who eats poorly and hates exercise; create a schedule for someone who wants a life; build a budget for someone who gets real joy from spending. The problem is, we don't want to be one of those people, so we continue to design strategies for a person we've never met.

Each of us has our authentic self and our desired self. The only way to get to the desired self is to start at the authentic self and do the work the authentic self doesn't want to do.

One of the problems with assessing present reality is that we can't embrace what we don't see. There is an old adage that goes, "You can't see the spinach in your own teeth." I'll bet when you hear yourself on a recording you think that that's not your real voice, that somehow you've been magically dubbed. Often, the same goes for present reality. That's why it's important to surround yourself with people who are willing to bring your attention to what you can't see about yourself. I believe that great leaders and highly effective people want to know what present reality is, but most of us want someone to validate our made-up version of ourselves.

People know which of their friends, co-workers, and relatives want to know the truth and which don't. Your job is to be the kind of person who wants to live the truth. Live your life based on what is real and true right now, not what you wish were true or think should be true.

What are the realities of your life that you avoid? Physical health, financial health, stress level, quality of your relationship, job satisfaction? Unless you start from the beginning, at a place grounded in reality, and unless you are in touch with *what is*, your chances of winning the game go down precipitously. If you are in denial or fantasy, or are out of touch with what is real, the rest of the rules won't matter much.

Rule #2 – Be Right About The Right Things

What's the population of Angola? I'm guessing you don't know, and neither do I; but how quickly could we find out? Probably in less than a minute. We live in an age of unprecedented access to information. There is absolutely no parallel in human history for what we are experiencing right now because of the Internet. While everyone knows change happens at a ridiculous pace, I don't think most people are really aware of the magnitude of what we are going through, or of one of the biggest dangers this presents. The danger I am talking about is a strange contradiction.

> **The easier access we have to information, the less informed people are becoming.**

To illustrate this point, here is a challenge for you. Turn on MSNBC, then Fox News, then CNN – for fifteen minutes each. Be careful, because you might have a stroke. They'll probably be talking about the same story but it will appear that it happened on three different planets. How can this be? Aren't these "news" organizations supposed to help us be more informed? Not anymore.

The news divisions of networks used to cost them money. They provided a service whose purpose was to inform the public and bolster the reputation of the network. Accuracy was something they prided themselves on. Then Ted Turner figured out that there was money in them thar' hills and founded CNN in order to make a profit. From then on, the nature of news has changed. Today, the main mission of news organizations is to make money through ratings and advertising; the focus is on how to get people to tune in. And it turns out, if people don't like what they hear, they change the channel. If I'm a liberal, why would I listen to Fox News rail against how awful President Obama is if instead I can just listen to MSNBC praise him endlessly? If I'm a conservative, why would I listen to MSNBC spell out how evil the conservatives are if I can just turn to Fox and have it made clear to me that liberals are the cause of all the problems in the world?

It used to be that we only had a few sources of information and newsrooms did this thing called journalism, where they at least made an attempt to be unbiased. It is very difficult to find someone still doing that today. Now, we have an almost unlimited amount of information sources, most of them presenting opinions as though they were facts. But boy, does our Emoter like this. You can now customize your information stream so that you don't have to hear anything the Emoter doesn't want to hear. What a country! You are motivated to have your Emoter feel good. Having the accuracy of your beliefs and perceptions challenged can be a very uncomfortable experience for the Emoter. As a result, most people watch the news to have their worldview validated, not confronted. The networks know this and program accordingly.

The problem is, the Emoter loves to be right. When you combine the Emoter's urge for rightness with a massive array of information to choose from, you unwittingly filter what you pay attention to down to what verifies your existing beliefs.

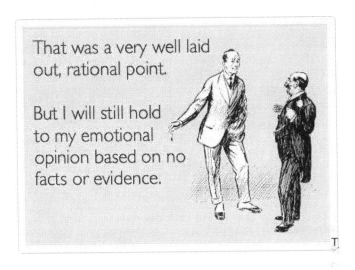

In his book, *The Information Diet: A Case for Conscious Consumption*, Clay Johnson does a great job of detailing what is going on with news today. One example he gives is of what Fox News does with stories on its website:

The AP's story "Economic Worries Pose New Snags for Obama" turned into "Obama Has a Big Problem with White Women." "Obama to Talk Economy, Not Politics, in Iowa" turned into "White House Insists Obama's Iowa Stop for Economy, Not 2012." And "Malaysia Police Slammed for Cattle-Branding Women" turned into "Malaysian Muslims Cattle-Brand Prostitutes."

Contrary to the popular belief on the left, Fox isn't evil, it just knows how to make money by taking advantage of people's Emoters. Don't blame Fox, blame our lack of understanding how we process information. MSNBC, The Huffington Post, The Drudge Report – the list goes on of others doing the same thing, although I think Fox is best at triggering the Emoter for profit.

The danger of this misinformation stream that we unwittingly digest, is that it supports us in feeling more self-righteous about our beliefs. If you put a bunch of liberals in a room together, they leave feeling more liberal. The same is true for conservatives. If all you hear is, "You're right, you're right, you're right," you end up believing you're right. Having never heard anything to contradict your beliefs, why would you change them?

One of the remedies Clay Johnson suggests is to get as close to the source as possible. Fox spends seventy-two percent of its operating budget on program expenses (things like on-air talent); MSNBC spends eighty-eight percent. That doesn't leave much money for field journalists. Instead, they rely on getting their stories from sources like the Associated Press, AOL, Reuters, and even bloggers. Then they spin it to feed their viewers what they know the viewers want to hear. As Johnson puts it:

> "The strategy is simple: it's cheaper to pay one media personality a two million dollar salary than it is to pay 100 journalists and analysts $40,000 a year. What's better, people like hearing their beliefs confirmed more than they like hearing the facts."

His last line spells out the need for this rule, which is "Be Right about the Right Things." I am not suggesting the fix is to try to let go of your desire to be right. That's not likely to succeed. Instead, we need to understand how strong this desire is, and use it to drive us to seek out better information. With better facts, you can be even MORE right, which the Emoter loves.

The skill you will need to develop in order to do this, is the ability to separate fact from opinion and knowledge from belief. The biggest problem with our information stream today, is people stating their beliefs as though they are facts.

You have to learn to be able to tell the difference and understand what you are hearing.

In my courses, I sometimes suggest a hypothetical exercise that goes like this: take a piece of paper and write down everything you think about global warming. There will likely be a variety of items like, "It's totally happening and is man-made" or "It's a natural cycle of the planet" or "It's hype ginned up by the liberal media," etc. Then I say, "What if I asked you to now take out a piece of paper and write down everything you *know*: not opinions, not beliefs – just facts, knowledge, and information." Most people would have a much shorter list on this page. It turns out that as humans, we need little or no information to form an opinion. To really consider how much you know, and compare it to how much you don't know, is a very humbling experience.

So the challenge I offer with this rule is to consciously decide what you want to be right about, and then dig for good information. Can you let in information that is different from what you already believe? How good are you at changing your mind?

Rule #3 – Own the Game

A very common practice for many people is to think, "If (they, she, he, it) were different, I'd be fine. If my parents were different, if my boss were different, if my spouse were different, if the world were different (you get the picture), I'd be fine." But the problem is, we don't get a choice about reality (see rule #1). People and situations have an annoying habit of being the way they are.

For example, let's say I believe I have a terrible boss. I could easily convince myself and the people around me that she/he is the problem, and I could gather enough evidence to prove that to be true. I think, "Anyone with half a brain can see it's not about me. I've done the research and I clearly see that she or he is the reason I'm not successful." But as soon as I am successful at proving that to myself and others, I give the game away, and in doing so I put the power of solution outside of me. More importantly, I put my success outside of me as well.

Giving the game away, allows me to stay in Passive Thinker. Since they are the problem, not me, I don't have to engage my Active Thinker to solve it. They need to change, not me. In our desire to prove we are not the problem, we give the game away. The strategy that works in life is to own the game, not the blame.

I'm not a big fan of positive thinking. I'm not trying to convince you that your boss, your spouse or the situation you are in is wonderful. They/she/he/it may be terrible. I'm saying that as a strategy, positive thinking by itself doesn't work. I'm a fan of effective thinking. Call the problem what it is, then get busy.

So instead of, "If they were different, I'd be fine." Or, "They are wonderful. This isn't a problem, it's an opportunity." Change it to, "Given they are the way they are, how can I get what I want?" As soon as you own the game, you have choice. You can't change reality; all you have are your choices of response to reality. The more you own the game, the more effective your responses become. When you think, "If they were different, I'd be fine," the only solution is waiting for them to change, which probably isn't going to happen. All you end up getting is better at resentment and frustration and using your Passive Thinker to come up with clever and creative ways to feel like a victim. Owning the game is not a comfortable choice; it's the most effective choice.

Rule #4 – Let the Future Be Your Guide

You will find that when you make damaging choices, that more often than not the image on the screen that the Emoter is responding to is based solely on the immediate consequences, not the future ones. Without the long and short term effects of your actions, the image is lacking all the facts.

For example, let's say you have a piece of cheesecake in front of you whose demise you are contemplating. With a focus on the short term, the Emoter's choices are:

1) Eat the cheesecake and feel happy.
2) Not eat the cheesecake - suffer and be deprived.

Hmmmm. Not a tough choice. But if the Thinker steps in and the image on the screen changes by adding in the future, the Emoter's response changes. Now the choice becomes:

1) Eat the cheesecake - feel good in the moment, then feel bad later because of the outcome.
2) Not eat the cheesecake - feel good later because of the outcome.
3) Eat the cheesecake - balance that with portion control and exercise; feel good now and later.

Now the scene is different for the Emoter. When you bring the future into the decision making process, you see different options.

The more time the Thinker spends in Active mode, the easier this rule becomes. I'll give you some ideas for how to keep the Thinker Active in the next Chapter.

Rule #5 – Life Happens Gradually, Then Suddenly

A character in an Ernest Hemingway book was once asked, "How did you go bankrupt?" The character replied, "Well, gradually, then suddenly." It turns out that almost everything in our lives happens this way.

I have to apologize to you, and probably the rest of the world, as I am partly to blame for the current horrible economy and housing crisis. In 2001, my wife and I relocated from Seattle to Albany, N.Y., where we would be closer to friends and family, live in a market with cheaper housing and less traffic, and be in a better location when traveling for work; at the time, I was spending most of my time on the east side of the Mississippi.

Shortly after settling there, we bought an old pickle factory. It was a funky old building in the middle of a residential neighborhood that was pretty much abandoned when we came across it. No, it did not smell like pickles; it hadn't been a pickle factory since the late nineteen-sixties, but we liked to call it our pickle factory anyway. We renovated it into a couple of apartments, as well as a very spacious and cool living area for us.

The way the loan worked was that we got the place for $60 thousand, then drew up plans and showed them to an appraiser who said, based on those plans, the finished property would be worth $145 thousand. We got a loan from the bank for $160 thousand, which was more than the place was worth! This was a mind-numbingly stupid loan. Fortunately, we didn't default on the loan but many others with similar loans did.

Why did they give us that loan? Because it wasn't much riskier than the loans they gave out the day before, the month before or even the year before. It was significantly riskier than the loans they gave out ten or twenty years earlier. This is how life tends to happen. The changes in the wrong direction happened so slowly and so gradually that most people didn't notice them until it was too late.

If you think about the results in your life, you'll probably have difficulty finding an example of something that didn't happen gradually then suddenly. A woman in one of Jim's courses once said, "I became overweight one Cheeto at a time." People work longer and longer hours with the "suddenly" perhaps being a relationship that fails. Graduating from school, career progress, and stress levels are all "gradually then suddenly" examples.

There is always a gradual that leads to a sudden, but sometimes we experience a sudden that had a gradual in which we had no participation. Maybe you're at a stoplight and someone rear-ends you. It's a sudden for you, but how the other person gradually got to the point of being a bad driver had nothing to do with you. For most of the results in your life though, you actively participate in the gradual that brings *suddens* about, for better or for worse.

Your finances, body, and lifestyle are all great examples of areas of your life that come about gradually, then suddenly. Contrary to popular belief, there is a limit to how fast the body can gain weight. And contrary to popular diet plans, there is a limit to how fast it should lose it. Over sixty percent of lottery winners go bankrupt afterwards; some eighty percent of people who do debt consolidation or bankruptcy end up deeper in debt. Most people who lose weight on a crash diet gain it back and then some. When we try to create the sudden without the gradual, the Robot rarely has the time to change, so the results don't last.

Here's an example. A woman approached me after a course and talked about her vision and plan for weight loss and getting in shape. She said, "I'm going to go to the gym three times a week!" I tried to help her embrace present reality by asking, "How often do you exercise now?" She said, not at all. She was going to go from nothing to twelve times a month. The Robot simply does not change that quickly without a major trauma, which means the only way she'll keep that plan up is for her Thinker to constantly override the Emoter. This is called will power and it won't last long.

I recommended that she go to the gym two, three, maybe four times in the first month. I asked how hard that would be. She said, "That would be easy!" You could see the excitement radiating from her Emoter. Then I said, "Great. After two or three months, when that feels like something you can maintain, add another day and so on, until a year or two from now you'll be going three times a week and then, "suddenly", you'll be there."

I'm not suggesting this would be the right way for everyone. You will have to learn how best to work with your Emoter so that you can gradually, then suddenly, change your Robot. More on working with the Emoter in the next chapter.

To win The Internal Game, you need to recognize that one of the keys to success is to remember that the secret is in the gradual. The Emoter wants the sudden to happen *right now*. It's going to be the Thinker's job to understand that the Robot changes gradually, not suddenly, so quick fix approaches are not going to be the answer.

Rule #6 – Build a Good Team

I once heard it said that we become the average of the five people we spend the most time with. My first thought was, "Man, you people gotta go." My second thought was, "I wonder if they are saying the same thing about me?" I now think it would be more accurate to say we become the average of the five people we are most influenced by.

Who are you influenced by? It might be the people you spend the most time with or it might be someone else. This also begs the question, how much are you influenced by others? When I first heard that expression more than fifteen years ago, I did what the speaker suggested and estimated the net worth of the five people I spent the most time with. It turned out that mine was right about the average of the five. Plus, they were all married like me and had similar interests. It was surprising how true the statement was for me at the time.

A friend once asked me to support him with some difficulties he was having with his marriage. He knew I had a successful and happy marriage, and was very well read on the subject, so I agreed. I gave him some books to read and we talked about what he had discovered. He was applying what he had learned very diligently, but after about three months he was getting frustrated with how things were going. I asked him who his wife got support from and he said her mother and sister who, between them, had seven divorces and were both single. He was building a better team; hers needed some work.

I think most people are passive when it comes to the topic of support. Rarely do we consciously do an inventory of the support we have available or how much we use it, but that is exactly what I am suggesting you do with this rule. What kind of team do you have supporting you and do you use it? Here are some thoughts:

- It has been suggested that we get no more than thirty percent of our support from our spouse. Many people think of their significant other as being responsible for much more than that. But when we lean on them that heavily, we put too much of a burden on the relationship and it can strain.

- Many people are more willing to give support than they are to ask for it. Is it easier for you to do something for a friend than it is to ask for something for yourself?

- Mentors are very good things to have. You may even have someone in your life who, if you asked them, would be happy to mentor you. You will probably also be surprised at how easy it is to find one; possibly it's someone who you don't currently know. Most people are honored to be asked.

- Mentors don't have to be your everything. You might have someone you know who is very good with money but horribly stressed out. Ask them to be a financial mentor and find someone else for stress.

The bottom line is that going it alone is simply harder than it needs to be. If you ask someone you feel is successful about the topic of support, most, if not all of them will point to a list of people who helped them get to where they are.

I'm not suggesting that you get rid of your friends. I'm suggesting that if your present support system is not getting you the results you want, you may need to do some recruiting to help balance it out or fill in some gaps. What does your team look like? Do you need to do some recruiting?

Rule #7 – Be in Service

This rule is about paying attention to the effect of your actions. Are you doing harm or are you adding value? The concept is simple; when we are being in service, our lives work better. The practice is often not so simple.

As an example, years ago I was teaching a course to a room full of nurses. I think nurses are great examples of people who give huge amounts of themselves to their jobs, often too much for their own health. I wanted to make the point that being in service to everyone is a good idea, and everyone includes themselves. What I got was an explosion of anger and negativity that I rarely experience in my courses.

What got this room full of very nice, very giving people so angry with me, was that being in service to everyone meant being in service to doctors. They did not like doctors. They did not want to serve doctors. They very much wanted to serve patients, but doctors – not so much. As I dug deeper into where the anger originated, I found that almost to a person, they felt that doctors disrespected them, dismissed them, and condescended to them. In short, doctors were not in service to them, so they did not want to be in service to doctors.

Some people in the room came around to seeing the point I was making, others did not. I was encouraging them to be in service to everyone, even if the service was not reciprocated. The nurses and doctors were both there to serve the patient. Isn't doing everything they can to help each other the best way to do that?

I felt their pain, and I think almost everyone can empathize with them. Why on earth would I want to be in service to someone I have such animosity towards? The answer is, because it is what is best for me. Of course a nurse is there to serve the doctor. Ideally, the doctor sees him or herself as being there to serve the nurses as well, but even if they don't, I wanted what was best for the nurses. For many nurses, being in service is what they are good at and what they enjoy. I didn't want the nurses to pull back from that just because the doctor was a jerk. The doctor may have deserved it but the nurses didn't.

This concept represents one of the biggest changes taking place in the world of management and leadership today. Jim and I spend an enormous amount of time convincing companies and leaders that one of the main jobs of a manager is to be in service to his or her employees. We get resistance to this because in old school thinking, it is the other way around.

In one of Jim's courses, someone once asked about Steve Jobs, who was known for being rough on those who worked for him. The person asked, "How come he was so successful if he was the way he was?" Jim replied, "Genius trumps jerk." He was so brilliant that people were willing to put up with treatment they didn't want, but most managers need their people's Emoters to want to work for them. So unless you are a genius, it's best to learn how to be in service to your people. It's probably a good idea, even if you are a genius, which I'm sure you are.

Just to be clear, don't discount your own needs to be in service. That only creates resentment, bitterness, and martyrdom. It's about how can you fill your needs while being in service to others. Great leaders and highly effective people experience the joy of true service, service from a place of strength and fullness.

When we give up our own needs to serve others, we become a caretaker. There is a big difference between being in service to others and being a caretaker. Caretaking is when I help others to my own detriment. The reality of caretaking is that we do it more for ourselves than for others. We do it because we want them to like us, to need us, or in order to feel valuable. In the end, caretaking someone doesn't help them, so if helping them is what I am truly after, I wouldn't do it. We caretake because our Emoters get something out of it in the moment, and the Passive Thinker is not pointing out the damage we are doing to both of us in the long term.

Why the word "serve" rather than "support?" Some of the nurses wanted to think of themselves as supporting the doctors but serving the patients. I'd say go with the word that works best for you but really challenge yourself as to why it does. For some people, the word feels like being less than or beneath the person you serve. I get that.

But the people I know with the strongest *in service* mindset don't feel inferior or even appear that way. I don't know anyone who lives this rule better than Jim, and I know few people who are as well respected as he is.

Summary

When you follow the rules of the game, you are more effective at creating the results you want. They are not laws though, because you don't have to follow them. Things just work better when you do.

Rule #1 – Embrace Present Reality
Rule #2 – Be Right about the Right Things
Rule #3 – Own the Game
Rule #4 – Let the Future be your Guide
Rule #5 – Life Happens Gradually, then Suddenly
Rule #6 – Build a Good Team
Rule #7 – Be in Service

Part Three

Winning the Game

8

Getting Your Groove Off

I read a study once, which stated that sixty-five percent of people who undergo heart bypass surgery don't change their lifestyles long term. What does it take to change? Apparently, the threat of death is not enough. Studies like this and many others strongly make the point that we are not good at creating new behaviors, even when we really need to.

This is the chapter where you will learn how to create new behaviors and break out of those ineffective, self-destructive, well-worn neural pathways in your brain, and create new and hopefully better ones! These grooves you've created in your Robot over many years are often deep and wide; changing them is going to take some work.

To review, the Robot is what gives rise to all your thoughts and emotions. You have the ability to override it but if you don't, your pre-programmed context, paradigm, beliefs, etc., will shape and form what you see, how you see it, and how you respond. In addition, your ability to override the Robot is limited, both in scope and duration. Given all of this, if you want to create a lasting change in your life, whether it's something tangible like financial or physical health or something intangible, like stress, you will have to change your Robot.

We've explored the inner workings of the mind and what drives us. Now it is time to put it all to work. I'll do my best to boil down the mountain of information, data, research, and experience from both mine and Jim's careers into one simple formula. Will this be a gross over-simplification of the human condition? Of course it will. Simple doesn't even begin to describe my work. Wait, that's not right.

What I mean to say is that humans are very complex creatures. One of the things Jim and I have in common is a strong desire to boil things down to make them as easy to understand and apply as possible. Therefore, our approach has just five variables. Each has some depth and complexity to be sure, but most, if not all of us, can remember to pay attention to five things. If you can master these five components, you will be able to create wonderful things in your life. If you look at your efforts that have failed in the past, you will likely find that one or more of these ingredients was missing.

To create a new program in the Robot, you must be motivated by something strong and meaningful. In order for that motivation to turn into a permanent pattern in the Robot, the Thinker has to be in Active mode, which means focusing on both the present and the future. The Emoter must be engaged in, or at least be willing to make the new behavior permanent. The necessary structure and environment to support the new action has to be present, and you have to do this for a long enough period of time.

<u>The Robot Reprogramming Formula</u>

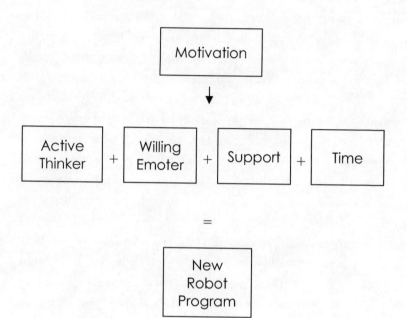

Motivation

The Robot is a stubborn character. It is designed for efficiency: doing what you have always done takes less effort. Consequently, to make a change that will override the Robot's built-in resistance is going to take a powerful motivator.

Americans do not lack motivation. We are one of the hardest working countries in the world. The average American works far more hours than people in almost every other modernized country.

If this is the case, why do so many people struggle to motivate themselves to make the changes they want to make? How can we be so motivated in some areas of our lives, yet feel completely flummoxed when it comes to making the changes we want in others?

It's because most people don't understand what really motivates them, so they end up being motivated by the wrong things. Because of this, we do the right things for the wrong reasons, or the wrong things for the right reasons. In order to do the right things for the right reasons, you're going to have to figure out the reasons. *Why* are you doing what you do? The answer is, the Emoter.

Every action you take, decision you make or behavior you choose is driven by one thing – the Emoter. You are motivated to please the Emoter. The problem is that you probably don't know how to do this. So you pick behaviors that you think will please the Emoter. The behaviors don't work, or you make decisions that do please the Emoter briefly but that may do damage later. In short, you need to learn how to please your Emoter in healthy and effective ways.

Motivation is about feeding the Emoter – and the Emoter must be fed. If the Emoter is not being fed, it will cast about for anything it believes will satisfy it as soon as possible. This is the root of destructive behaviors: feeding your Emoter in ways that wear off quickly and cause damage later.

> **An unfed and unhappy Emoter can be a dangerous thing.**

Let's start by looking at the most popular method that is used to feed the Emoter.

The DO – HAVE – BE Model

The DO – HAVE – BE model is an unconscious framework for how most Americans unwittingly live their lives. Here's how it works:

The DO is the way you spend your days: your job, marriage, hobbies, etc. The HAVE is all your stuff: your house, car, family, electronics, body, schedule, money, etc. The BE is the way you are supposed to feel as a result of all the DO-ing and HAVE-ing.

For example, in the area of health, you might exercise (DO) so you can lose weight (HAVE) so you will feel good about yourself (BE).

For wealth, you might save money (DO) so you can retire in comfort (HAVE) so you will be happy when you do (BE).

For stress, you might work long hours (DO) because you are supposed to have a busy schedule (HAVE) so you will be a good employee (BE). Or you pack your kids schedule full of activities (DO) so they will be well rounded and successful later (HAVE) so they will be happy (BE).

> ## The problem with the DO – HAVE – BE approach to life is that the BE you are hoping for usually doesn't arrive.

This is such a deep part of our conditioning that, as a nation, we DO more and HAVE more than any country in history. But we don't BE more. In other words, if DO – HAVE – BE worked, we'd be experiencing nearly endless bliss. Instead, when the BE that shows up isn't what we thought it would be or never even comes, we work harder at the DO and the HAVE because it's the only approach we know.

There are a ton of baby boomers waking up to the idea that all the DO-ing and HAVE-ing that they were supposed to do and have is not giving them the BE they wanted. They unconsciously followed this model and fell victim to its two *fatal flaws*, and the results are starting to show up.

Here's a quote from Danial Pink's *Drive*:

"In other words, in America alone, one hundred boomers turn sixty every thirteen minutes.

Every thirteen minutes another hundred people – members of the wealthiest and best-educated generation the world has ever known – begin reckoning with their mortality and asking deep questions about meaning, significance, and what they truly want.

One hundred people. Every thirteen minutes. Every hour. Of every day. Until 2024.

When the cold front of demographics meets the warm front of unrealized dreams, the result will be a thunderstorm of purpose the likes of which the world has never seen."

That's a whole lot of people wondering why the BE they thought would show up, hasn't.

We are motivated to please the Emoter, to feed the Emoter, and the DO – HAVE – BE approach is supposed to do that. When it doesn't, some of us try variations of the model in an attempt to find a method that works better.

For some people, especially in recent years, the HAVE – DO – BE approach is used. "If I won the lottery, I could HAVE anything I want, then I could DO anything I want, and *then* I would BE happy." I mentioned in Chapter 6 that we, as a nation, have started to worship HAVE-ing the American dream over achieving (DO-ing) the American dream. This makes the older generations crazy because they worship DO-ing. Neither works.

Some people just use the DO – BE approach. This is what creates workaholics. They don't have the BE, so the answer must be more DO-ing. They don't even care about the things they have, they just want to work, but they can't seem to DO enough.

Others try the HAVE – BE approach. Entitlement comes from the belief that you shouldn't have to DO anything; you should just get to HAVE what you want. This idea can lead to being a shopaholic or hoarder. They don't have the BE, so the answer must be to HAVE more, but they can't seem to HAVE enough.

You can never DO enough or HAVE enough; you can only BE enough.

Simply put, the DO – HAVE – BE approach is ineffective at creating the BE your Emoter desires. Without the BE, the Emoter is not fed and it starts to want things, which drives up your temptations. Those are the temptations behind the Never Enough Mindset. You do what you've been conditioned to do, which is more DO-ing and more HAVE-ing. That satisfies your temptations, but not enough. The answer to "not enough" feels like "more" – more DO-ing and HAVE-ing. This vicious circle is why America over-does everything but can't get enough. To break out of this cycle, you need a better way to create the BE your Emoter wants and needs.

The reason the DO – HAVE – BE model fails to produce the BE comes from its two *fatal flaws*, which are:

1) It uses extrinsic motivation.
2) It aims at the wrong target.

Flaw #1 – Extrinsic Motivation

Extrinsic is the technical term for external. The opposite is intrinsic, or internal. You are extrinsically motivated when your reason to act comes from outside of you. DO – HAVE – BE is an extrinsic approach because it is using the outside, the DO and the HAVE, as the source of motivation.

Extrinsic motivation is problematic because it is a victim approach to life, meaning the power lies outside you. As such, extrinsic motivation violates Rule #3 – Own the Game. If you are motivated by external forces, or hoping the external will fix the internal, you are not owning your game. You are at the mercy of the things you DO or the stuff you HAVE. They are in charge of your game. In other words, your life is running you, rather than you running your life.

Another problem with extrinsic motivation is that it tends to diminish or eliminate intrinsic motivation. The reason for this gets back to what we were talking about earlier: feeding the Emoter. The things you do for fun are the things you are intrinsically motivated to do. When you are reading a good book or engaged in your favorite hobby, you are motivated by the event itself. Your Emoter gets fed during the event. The *action* is what the Emoter thinks will make it happy.

When you are extrinsically motivated, your reason to act is not the event itself, but what you will get after the event. In other words, the Emoter doesn't get fed until the event is over. This is why the extrinsic tends to kill the intrinsic: because you care less about the behavior and more about the reward coming later. The *outcome* is what the Emoter thinks will make it happy so the actions matter less. The net effect is that you don't enjoy the ride along the way.

To summarize, the first flaw of the DO – HAVE – BE model is that it is an extrinsic approach. Extrinsic motivation puts the power of your life outside of you and simultaneously diminishes or eliminates the enjoyment of the action itself because you are motivated by the outcome, not the action.

Flaw #2 – Wrong Target

Motivation is about feeding the Emoter, and the second flaw with the DO – HAVE – BE model is that it uses a source of food that doesn't fulfill the Emoter's appetite. When you use this model, you are targeting either the DO or the HAVE. They are the wrong targets. You need to learn how to target the BE.

What does the Emoter eat? The Emoter can't DO anything. The things you DO are behaviors or actions that you perform; they are not what the Emoter eats. The same is true with HAVE. You don't feel what you HAVE, you feel what you *experience*. The Emoter doesn't feed on behaviors or possessions, it feeds on *experiences*. Only the BE can feed the Emoter and the BE is an *experience*.

Most people don't understand the difference between an action, an outcome, and an experience. Your Emoter wants experiences, but instead all you give it is actions or outcomes. The DO and the HAVE are the wrong targets because they are not Emoter food.

I want you to learn how to aim at the right target, and that target is the *experience* of life you desire. The BE is that *experience*, but with the DO – HAVE – BE approach, the *experience* you are after is a hopeful side effect of the way you live. The solution is to have the *experience* of life that you want be what your life is about; your actions and outcomes are there to support that experience.

The answer, I believe, is to learn how to use intrinsic motivation instead of extrinsic and to aim at the right target. You do this by using the BE – DO – HAVE approach. Let go of the mistaken belief that the problem with your life is the way you spend your days or the things you surround yourself with. Learn how to feed your Emoter by giving it what it truly wants: a rich and full experience of life.

> The secret to effective and lasting change is to be *intrinsically* motivated by the <u>experience</u> of life you desire; not actions, possessions or outcomes.

Experiential Motivation

> *"Martin Luther King, Jr. gave the "I Have a Dream" speech, not the "I Have a Plan" speech."* – From the 7th most watched TED.com video by Simon Sinek, author of *Start with Why: How Great Leaders Inspire Everyone to Take Action.*

Noel is a five-foot, eleven-inch, forty-year-old, stunningly attractive woman with inexplicably low standards in men, given she's my wife. We've been married for more than sixteen years.

Like many people in our country, Noel has struggled with her weight for years. She's been on almost every popular diet and has experienced the up and down cycle that is the common result of that method. Then, in February 2012, she used a different approach. She lost thirty-six pounds in six months and has kept if off for the last seven. This is the first time she has hit her weight loss goal and the first time she has maintained a constant weight for longer than a month or two.

During the time she was losing weight, her mother asked her, "What size do you want to get down to?" Noel replied, "It's not really about a size. I just want to feel different." When I asked her what was different about this time as compared to her prior efforts, she said, "I just didn't want to feel old and unattractive."

This is a great example of what it means to be experientially motivated. What Noel did was to use the BE, or the *experience* of life she wants, as her driving force. She didn't think any specific behavior or outcome was going to change her. It was a BE – DO – HAVE approach.

In the next chapter, you will hear the stories of three other people who have created lasting change in their lives. When I asked them the question, "What motivated you?" none of them could put it into exact words, but they all had a very clear sense of it. They knew the *experience* they wanted: their BE, or their *why*, and it drove them. They said things like, "I just didn't want to feel that way." Or, "That was not who I wanted to be." By getting clear on the experience they were missing in their lives, they knew the experience they wanted to create.

They struggled to put clear words to the experience they wanted because it was not something tangible. We think we want tangible things, like the DOs and the HAVEs, but we don't. We want the BE. The BE is harder to explain because it happens deep inside you. I'm going to make it easier for you to find it and explain it. I'm going to help you find the words, but what matters most is your sense of it. The words will help, but as you can see from Noel's example and the others to come, as long as you can feel it, it can drive you.

I'm going to give you two methods to help you figure out your desired experience that will drive the changes you want to make:

Clarifying Your Desired Experience - Method #1

Method #1 goes like this: ask yourself *why?* Then keep asking yourself why until you are clear on the experience you want, not a behavior you want to force yourself to DO, or a tangible end result you want to HAVE.

For example, let's say you want to exercise three times a week. The reason so many people struggle to get this behavior programmed into their Robot is that they don't know *why* they really want to do this. If you were to ask yourself *why* you want to exercise, you might say, "to lose weight." But *why* do you want to lose weight? Do you want to feel a sense of achievement, look more attractive, be a good role model, enjoy a longer life, radiate more energy or perhaps something else? These answers are not actions you DO or something tangible to HAVE, they are the true experience of life you are after.

When you have clarity of the experience you want, it becomes fuel for the Emoter. It gives the Emoter what it wants while NOT making it dependent on the behavior. *The experience drives the behavior, not the behavior giving you the experience.*

To finish the exercise example, let's say the experience you are after is a sense of achievement, to feel attractive, and to be a role model for your kids. These are not things you HAVE, they are experiences. They are not anything you can put in your hands or quantify; you can only feel them. Achievement, feeling attractive, and being a role model are the BE, or the *why*. Exercising three times per week is the DO. A physically fit body is the HAVE.

In Noel's case, she wanted to feel different more than she wanted to look different. It wasn't about the way she looked; it wasn't about her size or her weight; it was about the experience of life she wanted to feel.

When you target actions or outcomes, once they have come and gone, any benefit you get from them goes as well.

You have the HAVE, and that's it. Now you're supposed to be happy. The BE came from the end, so it will be short lived. If you target goals or end results, your happiness is tied to them. If and when the end brings happiness, it doesn't last long. When it wears off, it will feel like it wasn't enough. With the experience, there are no ends. Don't aim for an end, aim for a different way of being.

Notice that with experience as the motivator, there are nearly endless options for the DO and the HAVE that allow you to feel the experience. In other words, knowing the experience you are after, you can create it in many ways while the experience motivates you to exercise.

Keep asking yourself *why* until you discover the core driving experience you are after; the behaviors that flow from that are what you want to imbed into your Robot. When that happens, your Robot will automatically create that experience for you.

You do this already. You have many behaviors programmed into your Robot that give you an enjoyable experience and don't cause damage down the road. This is about learning how to insert a new one, or replacing the ones that are causing damage.

Let's consider stress. Why do you want less stress? "Well, because I don't want to feel stress." It is very difficult to just eliminate something, especially when it's a symptom and not the problem. What works better is to replace what you are trying to get rid of with what you want. Do you want to experience more quality time with your kids? Do you want more peace or balance in your life? Pick something that you can move toward, not away from. Stress is often a side effect of your struggle to achieve a desired experience or, if you already have it, to keep it from disappearing.

Let's consider financial health. Why do you want it? Do you want to feel freedom and/or security? Do you want to be able to contribute to others? What's the experience you are after?

Getting clear about your driving experience can sometimes be as easy as asking yourself *why* enough times and then figuring it out. At other times, it will take more work than that. It could take digging into this question of *why* over a period of time. My challenge to you is to keep doing that digging until you find the clarity you need. Once you have it, get busy creating your world, rather than reacting to the world around you.

Two more quick thoughts: first, it does need to be specific enough that you can get to work on it. "Do Better" or "Be Happy" are too broad. Second, don't let life create your desired experience for you. Many people wait for a crisis before finding clarity. They get really sick, go through bankruptcy, get divorced, etc. Make a clear choice before the emergency comes.

Clarifying Your Desired Experience – Method #2

The genesis of real change comes when you recognize that the core experiences of your present life are not what you want them to be. It doesn't work to aim at, and hope to be motivated by, a new behavior; the fact is that you don't really want that behavior. If you did, you'd already be doing it. You want what you hope that behavior will do for you. It's the experience that you really want, and that's what will motivate you.

With the first method, I challenged you to dig underneath the actions and outcomes that you think you want, in order to discover the real experience of life you are after.

With method #2, I'll give you a more direct approach to figuring out that experience.

I'm going to give you a list of core experiences that drive everyone; your task is to personalize and tailor the list to fit your unique Emoter makeup. You may find some similarities between what you discovered with Method #1 and this list. In fact, looking at the experiences on this list may help you complete your answer to the *why* question from Method #1. But they don't have to match.

While your Emoter is unique to you, it also has some things in common with others. In fact, I believe there are some very deep intrinsic drives that all of us share. Your Emoter wants and needs certain experiences in order to feel fulfilled.

While this framework is true for everyone, it is not completely accurate for anyone. You will have to take it and make it your own. Personalize it so that it fits your Emoter.

Because these are the most basic and universal experiences that motivate your Emoter, I have named them the Emotivators. Your Emoter needs, and will find a way, to experience these Emotivators, so much so that they will drive you to do destructive things if you don't create them with constructive methods. These are the BE that your Emoter wants to be fed with.

Emotivators

Safety – The need to know that you are safe. You have a basic human drive to know that you will have food, water, shelter, security, etc. If this need is not met, none of the other Emotivators will matter. This need trumps all others. These are your survival needs.

If you can't feed yourself or your family, if you live in unsafe surroundings and have no home, this need is not met and striving to meet it will consume your thoughts and feelings – as it should. Interestingly, there are some people whose safety need is met but they still don't *feel* as though it is. This could show up as an inability to trust, extreme fear-based decision-making or even paranoia.

Pleasure – The enjoyment of the physical senses. The way that you connect with the world around you is through your senses: taste, touch, smell, sight, and sound. This is the most basic way in which you experience and enjoy the world around you.

Acceptance – The experience of being valued and valuable. Everyone needs to feel love; acceptance is the root experience of love. Self-acceptance trumps acceptance from others.
- Similar experiences: Recognition, Being the Center of Attention, Being Impressive, Belonging, Acknowledgement, Being Seen/Noticed, Being the Best, Feeling Attractive.

Independence – The experience of being different from the tribe, being an individual, and believing you can survive on your own.
- Similar experiences: Freedom, Autonomy, Uniqueness, Self-Determination, Being Special, Variety.

Contribution – The experience of adding value to others or the world.

- Similar experiences: Nurturing, Adding Value to a Cause Greater than Yourself, Making a Difference, Purpose.

Accomplishment – The need to feel you can do something. In order to feel all is right with the world, your Emoter must have a sense that it can get something done.
- Similar experiences: Mastery, Challenge, Achievement, Creativity, Order from Chaos, Organizing, Problem Solving.

Knowledge – The experience of having knowledge or the experience of acquiring it. Your Emoter likes to know that it knows things or can figure things out. Some people are driven more by having the knowledge while others are more driven by its acquisition.
- Similar experiences: Discovery, Insight, Wisdom, Learning, Innovation, Problem Solving, Creativity.

Notice a couple of things. I've listed some similar experiences under each Emotivator but the name for the Emotivator might be all you need. If that word really seems to resonate with your Emoter, you've got it. Some, like Creativity, are listed under more than one Emotivator. It just depends on what that experience does for you. This is also not a complete list. If you find an experience that really charges your Emoter, great – work with that. Very likely though, anything you come up with will connect back to one of these core drivers. Lastly, you could have two or more experiences that are about one Emotivator. I have two different ways I experience Acceptance. Your complete list does not have to match a particular number.

Your challenge is to look at each of these experiences and see if you can identify how it manifests in you. While I believe each of us finds a way to experience these Emotivators, the way in which you experience them is unique to you. For example, I know that my Emoter loves the experience of wisdom, challenge, nurturing, variety, being the center of attention, and feeling impressive. You can see how they fit into each category. For the last two, I don't really think about Acceptance but I know that that is how Acceptance shows up for me. There are not many rules here. Find what works for you.

Pick any of these Emotivators and try to imagine a life in which you never have that experience. I think it would be hard to do. In fact, you can probably think of someone who has an excessive and almost screaming need for one of these experiences. That comes from not fully having the experience, so they overcompensate for it. Let's look at some examples of how these experiences can show up, both constructively and destructively.

Constructive Methods: Both Jim and I have variety as one of our Emotivators. That is a big part of why we enjoy our careers. We work in different companies, in different parts of the country, and sometimes different countries on a regular basis. Every week is different from the last. A construction worker could experience accomplishment and contribution in their work. A scientist who publishes their work, could experience discovery and recognition. A customer service representative could be driven by nurturing and problem solving.

Destructive Methods: Someone with an excessive need to be right might be trying to experience knowledge and acceptance. A person obsessed with how they look could also be driven by a lack of acceptance. Codependent or caretaking behavior is often driven by a combination of a lack of self-acceptance and contribution. Over-eating, over-spending, over-scheduling, gossip, negativity: the list of the destructive ways we can go about satisfying our Emotivators is a long one.

Remember, all motivation is about feeding the Emoter. The Emotivators are the foundation of your Emoter's food pyramid. With time and attention, you will be able to see your Emotivators showing up in almost every aspect of your life. Clairty about how they show up will give you a much more effective handle on creating fulfillment and happiness.

Motivation Summary

You need motivation that is strong enough to drive behaviors that are not already programmed into the Robot. Your brain resists new behaviors because they take too much effort. As a result, this motivation has to be powerful. The most powerful motivator there is, is experience. Experiential motivation is the driver of real and lasting change.

The DO – HAVE – BE Model

- You are conditioned to believe that the right DO-ing and the right HAVE-ing will give you the experience of life you want. They usually don't.
- Actions are things you DO; things are what you HAVE; the experience we have as a result of these two is the BE.
- The BE – DO – HAVE approach works better and is about having the experience of life you desire drive your actions.

- Flaw #1 of the DO – HAVE – BE model is that it uses extrinsic motivation, meaning that you are motivated by outside influences. It is based on the belief that the outside will fix the inside.
- Flaw #2 is that it aims at the wrong target. This model targets behaviors and outcomes, both of which are finite. When you tie your happiness to behaviors and outcomes, your happiness ends when the behaviors and outcomes do. The right target is the experience of life you desire.

Experience as a Motivator

- The first method for discovering your motivating experience is to look at what you want to DO or HAVE and ask yourself *why?* Keep asking why until you get down to the core experience you are seeking, and make that your focus, not a behavior or outcome.
- The second method involves taking the list of Emotivators, which are universal driving experiences, and customizing it to your Emoter. You can then use that list to drive the changes you seek.

Active Thinker

The most critical part of this equation, and arguably the most important skill to develop in life, is getting your Thinker into Active mode. It has certainly been the most difficult part of my own journey in understanding what it takes to create real change. Master this step and you will be in rare company; most people can't tell the difference between Active and Passive Thinker states.

You don't require an Active Thinker in order to change but you do need it for effective change. With a Passive Thinker, the Emoter constantly drives you to change, just not necessarily for the better. You want the changes you experience to be intentional and helpful. To do this, you have to put the Thinker in charge. Being in charge doesn't mean being a dictator, it means being a collaborator, orchestrator, and leader. It's about having the Thinker use the best strengths of both the Emoter and the Robot to create a good future, and to enjoy the ride along the way.

The Active Thinker in Action

The easiest visual for understanding how the Active Thinker works is to imagine the Thinker holding the present in its left hand and the future in its right. Let's look at debt as an example. If your left hand holds "lots of debt" and your right hand holds "debt free," the Emoter gets very uncomfortable and tells the Thinker to drop one of them. The bigger the difference between the two, the louder the Emoter screams.

It is crucial to have a core driving experience that your Emoter wants and needs, because that experience is the glue that holds the left and right hand together. Without that aid, the Thinker just won't be strong enough to hold onto both of them.

You are at your best when the present and the future are linked together to create your experience of life. If you only hold onto the present, your thinking might sound like: "Why on earth would I eat broccoli instead of chocolate?" Or, "Why wait to have something I want later when I can have something I want now?" Or, "Say yes to everything, as long as saying yes feels good." If now is all you see, it is the only source of your experience.

If you only hold onto the future, then the future is the only source of your experience. The Emoter will not ignore what it is currently feeling for long, so you have to force yourself to keep moving for the sake of what might come later.

The people who have mastered those healthy behaviors you want for yourself, feel the benefit of the future they are creating while they create it. It's not misery now for the sake of later or misery later for the sake of now. When you know the experience that is driving you, you can experience it all along the way, both now and later.

For example, someone might say, "Wow, it feels good to eat healthy." It does feel good to eat right and exercise when you feel what it is doing for you. The person who might say this, is eating that way because their Emoter is having the experience of life it desires right then and there in addition to later.

"I love saving money." For the person saying this, it's true, because their future is connected to their present.

"I can't say yes to that because it will fill my schedule to overflowing. I love feeling like I have time." Again, the future is connected to the present.

These examples are of people who have already programmed their Robot with the present and future glued together. They have their desired experience even when their Thinker is in Passive mode. You do not – not yet. Your Thinker has to be in Active mode. It will have to hold onto the present and the future and keep a focus on the experience your Emoter wants as the glue to keep them together long enough for the glue to dry. When the glue dries, the Robot can take it from there.

What it will take to get your Thinker into Active mode varies from person to person. I have some suggestions that can help but these approaches don't work identically for all people. You will have to try different things to learn what works best for you. The most critical thing to remember is that if the Robot is in charge, it will not change itself. You must keep the Thinker Active long enough for the Robot to be re-wired. What follows are methods and strategies for getting into Active Thinker mode and for building a stronger Thinker with more endurance.

Manage the Screen

First you have to have a firm grip on present reality. Grab onto it with your left hand and hold on tight. You do this by using Rules 1, 2, and 3 all at the same time. Here is how each applies:

Rule #1 – Embrace Present Reality: If the Emoter doesn't like what is real and true right now, it tends to avoid or ignore it and the Robot will help by just tuning things out. What you are doing here is telling yourself the truth about what is going on. How stressed are you? What is your net worth? How healthy are you? You are not going to be successful at changing your Robot if you are out of touch with the current state of your life. This might be a cold, hard wakeup call. What is the present truth of your life? This rule is about examining and challenging your *awareness* of what is going on right now.

Rule #2 – Be Right about the Right Things: We all like to be right; this is about being clear about how that desire affects you. You will never lose your need to be right. The trick is to be right about the right things. This is about knowing the difference between facts and opinion, between knowledge and belief. This rule is about examining and challenging the *accuracy* of your view of reality.

Rule #3 – Own the Game: If current reality is not something you like or want, you tend to find something or someone else to blame. This is the essence of being in a victim state of mind. The Passive Thinker gets busy finding ways to justify that, "It's not my fault, I don't deserve this, it's not fair, etc." The Active Thinker simply recognizes that what is, is. Like it or not, this is what is true right now. This rule is about examining and challenging your *ownership* of reality.

> **You want to be *aware* of what is real,
> have an *accurate* take on it,
> and *own* it, good or bad.**

You accomplish this by "managing the screen." Let's review from the Robot Chapter the concept of the screen.

The Robot filters through the massive amounts of information you take in, decides what to ignore and what to pay attention to, assigns meaning to that, and puts it on the screen. Both the Thinker and the Emoter use this interpretation and tend to assume it is accurate and true.

For example, when I was in my twenties, I fell prey to the "No Interest for Six Months" credit card offers that arrived almost daily. My Emoter loved the look of them. I would think, "Wow, this is great. Of course I'm going to pay off my credit card debt but in the meantime, I can avoid paying any interest and I'll be debt free sooner!" My Passive Thinker went right along with it.

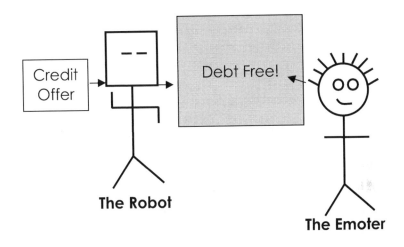

An Active Thinker would have looked at these offers very differently and done what those who are good with money do: throw them away. I obviously was not good at managing credit cards because I had already accumulated credit card debt. The net effect of another card was more debt. An Active Thinker would see this. Those of you who are good with money, or at least not using credit cards, think, "Duh, how obvious." But at the time, I didn't see it, and I had to learn to manage my screen before I could notice the truth.

What was the reality I would have found had I *Embraced Present Reality*? That I was in debt, bad at managing it, and continuing to accumulate more. Instead, what I told myself was, "I'll be out of debt in no time, nothing to worry about."

What was I being right about? That paying less interest would get me out of debt sooner. The problem was that, to me, this made sense. There was real logic to it. This often happens when we are not paying attention to the *Be Right about the Right Things* rule. We take something that has some truth and validity to it and use it to ignore other realities.

Was I *Owning the Game?* The ways we go into victim and put other people or other things in charge of our lives are many and varied. In this case, I was letting the marketing geniuses at the credit card companies run my screen rather than running it myself. I was letting myself be a victim of marketing.

When I see credit card offers now, my Emoter has a very deep and tangible negative response to them. I see them as doing me harm. It took a lot of work for me to change my emotional response. I didn't use will power to force myself to avoid getting another credit card. Instead, I used my Thinker to override and manage the image on the screen.

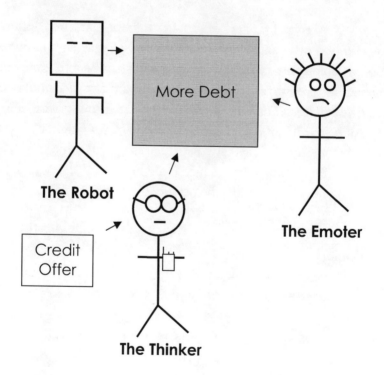

In the area of your life that you would like to change, your Robot's interpretations of the world are not working. If they were, you'd be getting the results you want. Your Robot might perceive stress when there is none, believe food will do something for you that it can't, or think spending or having something different will fill up an empty space inside.

The first step toward reprogramming the Robot is to question and challenge its interpretation of the world, which is what the screen is. A huge part of staying in Active Thinker is to be constantly curious. Why is that on your screen? Why are you seeing it that way? Why are you interpreting the situation this way? Who is running your perceptions and emotions? It is essential to have the humility to understand that just because you believe something, that doesn't mean it's true. It's about being willing to alter how you see the world.

My example may or may not resonate with you, so you might have to find a different one. I promise you, there are images and impressions being projected on your screen that are not working for you. No one has a perfectly programmed Robot. To change your Robot, you will have to catch and override the faulty programming. Again, three more case studies to follow in the next chapter.

Track the Future

In your right hand you need to hold onto the future. This is where you apply Rule #4 – Let the Future Be Your Guide. This is about having a picture of the future you want to create, and a way of tracking your progress towards it. Figure out the DO and the HAVE in BE – DO – HAVE. The HAVE is the future you want to create; the DO is the actions steps or behaviors that will lead you there.

I think the reason so many people set goals they never achieve is that they think the goal and/or vision will motivate them. They won't. That's not their job.

The job of a **vision** is to act as a target to aim at when making decisions. It is an outcome or a HAVE.

The job of a **goal** is to track progress along the way towards that vision and is also a HAVE.

A **plan** is the behaviors you choose that will produce the goals or vision and are actions or the DO.

Your **experience** is the reason behind all of these and is what you feel more and more as you move along the path. It is the BE.

Part of the job of the Active Thinker is to pay attention to the future you are moving towards and to make sure your experience shows up along the way.

Once they are clear on what their desired experience is, some people find they already feel it with the DOs and the HAVEs that exist at present. With better clarity on the experience you are after, you can experience it in your job, time with kids, family, or friends, the body you already have, your home, etc. The experience can help you enjoy what you already have. Most, if not all of your life is probably enough as it is. If that is the case, tracking the future is about making sure you are on a good course to keep things working.

Sometimes though, you will have to make some changes to your DO. If that is the case, the new plan might involve the use of some goals along the way. However, I want to point out two potential problems with goals.

First, we often confuse the work of choosing the goal with the work of getting the goal. For example, I used to sit down two or three times a year and take a hard look at my financial picture. Then I would craft a very detailed plan for getting out of debt with a month by month budget. My Emoter would feel, "Whew. That was tough, but boy did I do some good work there. Now I'm really on top of things." I rarely made it past the first month of the plan.

Second, goals can take the focus off present reality. You can probably think of a time at work when the focus on achieving a goal became the only thing that mattered. Anyone who pointed out problems that occurred along the way was labeled a negative naysayer. Notice that both these problems with goals are what a Passive Thinker does. In Active Thinker, we don't lose our focus on what is going on right now or the future we are creating; we keep one hand on each.

To put it another way, when the Emoter is in charge and the Thinker is in passive mode, our focus is usually on right now and we ignore the future. When the Emoter goes into goal setting with a Passive Thinker, our focus is on the future and we ignore right now. Active Thinker goal setting is when we are focused on right now AND the future. Ignoring either is what gets us into trouble. The Emoter clouds the reality of the future and the present.

The most critical part of this is to pay attention to the present while tracking the future you are creating. When you combine these two with the experience you chose, you will usually be able to tell if a step is a good idea or not. But in some cases, you will need to pick some goals to help plot the course along the way.

When you have a good picture of the future you want to create combined with a plan for getting there, and then constantly track present reality, you have an Active Thinker in charge. So what's your plan for creating your experience? How much work do you have to do to figure that out?

Get Out of Your Comfort Zone

Did you know that roughly seventy percent of lottery winners squander away their winnings in just a few years, or that most people who lose weight on a diet gain it back and then some? How about that most people who go through debt consolidation end up deeper in debt? Why is this? They got out of their comfort zone and found a way back in.

The comfort zone is the region in which your Robot customarily operates. Once you step outside of those bounds and leave that familiar space, the Robot starts sounding alarms. When the Emoter hears those alarms, it gets unhappy, and priority number one is getting those alarms to stop so the Emoter can feel better. The Passive Thinker then gets busy finding a way to make the Emoter happy again, and getting back into the comfort zone is usually the shortest path.

The only long-term solution that works is to change your comfort zone. That is essentially what we are doing with reprogramming the Robot. However, when you are outside your comfort zone, you have to have an Active Thinker that overrides and quiets the alarms so the Emoter doesn't have temper tantrums.

There is a benefit to being outside your comfort zone: the Robot can't be in charge because it has no programming for this foreign terrain. The Thinker will either attempt to get back to the familiar or it will work to manage the new behaviors required to operate in this unfamiliar terrain. Therefore, a good strategy for getting the Thinker into active mode is to simply leave your comfort zone, and then work to stay there until the Robot adjusts.

A simple strategy for leaving your comfort zone is to do things in ways you are not accustomed to: drive to work a different way; rearrange your desk, kitchen or house; try using your left hand instead of your right or right instead of left. Anytime you behave in a new way, you take the action away from the Robot and give it to the Thinker. While these may seem like trivial things, once the Thinker is awake and Active, you will notice that behaviors in other areas become easier to give to the Thinker.

For example, I've been a professional speaker now for more than seventeen years; being in front of people is very much within my comfort zone. A little while back, I took an Improv class. I did it because it sounded like fun (I'm weird that way), I thought it might add something positive to my presentations and, being in the middle of writing this book, I thought it would inspire creativity. What I did not expect was to find that it was out of my comfort zone. While being on stage wasn't, not having a script or talking points to follow, was.

I was surprised by a couple of things. First, even though my Emoter was enjoying it, I found myself wondering when it would be over, questioning why I was doing this, mentally discounting the other students to feel less bad by comparison, and just generally looking for a way out. I could actually feel the Robot sounding alarms that were almost overriding my Emoter having fun and my Thinker staying Active. I had to consciously work to stay in active mode and to keep engaged in the activity.

Second, I found that while I was out of my comfort zone, other parts of my life looked different. I was looking at them with the Thinker, not the Robot. Challenges felt easier. I had a more upbeat and positive attitude, and I more easily motivated myself to do things I was avoiding. These are all symptoms of an Active Thinker; I just didn't expect them to show up because I took an Improv class.

Now I'm not suggesting you go and take an Improv class, unless that sounds like fun to your Emoter. I am suggesting that if you want to create change in any area of your life, pick something that is outside your comfort zone that your Robot doesn't have completely figured out, and go for it, even if it has nothing to do with your desired area of focus.

Join Toastmasters; take a rock climbing course; do some charity work. Use the criteria that it has to be something your Robot can't handle on its own, and it has to be something that will charge your Emoter. The Emoter wants to do it, has some real energy about it, and is maybe even a little scared of it.

Build a Stronger Thinker

Your brain is like a muscle. Not in the literal sense, since the cells don't flex or contract, but figuratively, because the more you use the cells, the stronger they get.

More and more studies in the growing field of neuroplasticity show that we can actually grow new brain cells, and build better and stronger Thinkers. Here is a quote from Lumosity.com's site, which I'll talk more about in a minute:

"The Advanced Cognitive Training for Independent and Vital Elderly (ACTIVE) study was a large, randomized, controlled trial testing the effects of three kinds of cognitive training (Ball, et al., 2002). The 2,832 participants underwent approximately 10 one-hour sessions of training over about six weeks. This NIH-funded trial has produced a number of interesting results. Unsurprisingly, participants in all groups learned to perform the training tasks more efficiently. What was more impressive was that the effects of the training transferred to measures of real-world function. These functional benefits were observed five years after training was completed, indicating that the benefits were sustained for a substantial period of time (Willis, et al., 2006). The ACTIVE study demonstrates that cognitive training can have highly beneficial real-world benefits for seniors."

If you are interested, the site has more research findings. Lumosity is a site devoted to mental gymnastics. Founded and supported by real, credentialed researchers and scientists in the field, it features a collection of fun-to-play games that build a better Thinker. In their own words:

"Doctors and scientists have studied the brain for hundreds of years, marveling at its ability to acquire new knowledge late into life. Until recently, the scientific community believed that learning happened by changing the strength of neural connections. This idea stemmed from the belief that the structure and organization of the brain did not change much after childhood.

Over the last few decades, however, researchers have discovered that the brain can fundamentally reorganize itself when confronted with new challenges, and that this can occur regardless of age. Evidence suggests that the brain, when given the right exercise, can actually reshape itself to become more efficient. This ability, known by scientists as "neuroplasticity," has far-reaching consequences. Neuroscientists and researchers are continuously discovering new ways for leveraging neuroplasticity to improve the brain's health and performance."

I'm a fan of the site and have been using it to build my own better Thinker. I actually use it as a warm-up when I'm writing and I can feel the difference when I do. Here are some other strategies for exercising and growing your Thinker:

<u>Exercise</u> - According to the Alzheimer's Research & Prevention Foundation, physical exercise reduces your risk of developing Alzheimer's disease by fifty percent. Basically, Alzheimer's is a result of the Thinker and the Robot breaking down. Both get stronger with exercise.

<u>Use It</u> – Sudoku, crossword puzzles, anything that involves problem solving, activates your Thinker. The more you use it, the stronger it gets. However, if the Robot can do the action, it is not strengthening your Thinker.

<u>Keep Your Advice To Yourself</u> – Most people love giving advice. One study watched the brains of people solving a problem and found that their Frontal Cortex or Thinker, was very active. But when they gave them advice on how to solve the problem, the Thinker went quiet and the Robot got active trying to remember what had been said.

When we give advice, we turn off the other person's Thinker. When we seek advice, rather than working out the problem, we turn off our Thinker. What works better is to ask questions of someone seeking advice, or use brainstorming or collaboration if you want help from others. I'm not suggesting you have to solve all your problems on your own, just don't turn your Thinker off when borrowing others people's Thinkers; don't let them do your thinking for you.

Meditation/Prayer – Evidence is building to show that meditation, and, for some, prayer builds a stronger thinker. Both provide an opportunity to slow down, clear the mind, become aware of the moment, and hold a clear picture of what you want to create. The net effect is to stimulate the frontal cortex. There have even been brain scans done of an experienced meditator that show increased activity in their frontal cortex during meditation. The more you use it, the stronger it becomes.

Active Thinker Summary

The primary job of an Active Thinker is to be in touch with present reality and to track the future you are creating. Some tips for helping you do this:

Manage Your Screen
- *Embrace Present Reality* by telling yourself the truth about what the current state of your life is.
- *Be Right about the Right Things* by recognizing that you want to be right, and consciously deciding what you will base that on: knowledge or opinion.
- *Own the Game* by letting go of blaming yourself or others, or the notion of what is fair. What is, is. Be in charge of what goes on your screen and don't let others run your screen for you.

<u>Track the Future</u>
- Your desired experience acts as your guide for decision-making. It gives you direction and a way to track progress.
- Goals are often helpful for adding clarity and for measuring progress. Do you need some goals to help chart your course? Don't let the goals become more important than either the experience or present reality.

<u>Get Out of Your Comfort Zone</u>
- Try something new. Pick something that charges your Emoter, and that your Robot doesn't know how to do.

<u>Build a Stronger Thinker</u>
- Your Thinker grows stronger through mental exercises, physical exercise, meditation or prayer, and even through changing how you give and use advice.

Willing Emoter

Your destructive actions are attempts to please the Emoter. They are certainly not about logic. By "Willing Emoter" I mean that the action or behavior that the Active Thinker has chosen is one the Emoter either loves, likes or is at least willing to do. The Emoter doesn't have to love it, although it helps, but as long as it is not fighting against it or neutral about it, you will have the energy and motivation necessary to act. In short, you need to find a way to please the Emoter that isn't destructive.

When the Emoter is willing to do what you want, it is significantly easier to keep the Thinker Active. If the Emoter is unhappy or checked out for long enough, it will wrestle the wheel of the car away from even the strongest Thinker. This section is about how to keep the Emoter willing so it will be happy to ride shotgun. The Emoter does not mind having your internal adult in charge, as long as it is in favor of the direction you're heading.

Making the Emoter willing to do something it doesn't want to do can be tricky – but not as tricky as you might think. We all struggle with our Emoter when trying to create change but most of us are not conscious of the effort. You are already ahead of the pack because you have an understanding of the Internal Game. You are aware of the fight you're engaged in; others are battling blind.

What follows is a list of ideas that help. I wish I could just say, "Here, this is the way to work with your Emoter," but I can't. Your Emoter is unique to you and as such, your path to working with your Emoter will have to be as well. Try some or all of these suggestions and see which work best. If you come up with something that works better, let me know; I'd love to hear about it.

Honor the Emoter

One of the main aims of this book is to help you understand that your Emoter exists. Society constantly gives you messages that you shouldn't even have an Emoter. Americans tend to see emotions as a weakness. As a result, we try to ignore or suppress the Emoter when we feel something we don't want to. In many cases, we suppress the Emoter even when we feel good. Do you ever tell yourself, "Things are going too good; better watch out?"

The most crucial lesson to learn about creating a willing Emoter is to acknowledge that it exists, and to honor whatever the Emoter is feeling, good or bad. Instead, we try to tell ourselves that we shouldn't feel that way. "Shoulds" don't work.

You feel what you are feeling for a good reason. You might never figure out what that reason is, but at some point in the past your Robot got programmed in such a way that you are feeling the emotions you are experiencing now. Trust that there was a good reason for it, and that you have to do some updating because the programming that resulted no longer applies.

You can honor, respect, and love yourself the way you are and still understand that you need to make some changes. The problem is that you have been conditioned to drive yourself with shame and non-acceptance. I want you to use self-compassion, education, and experiential motivation instead.

How Much is Enough?

I think at times in this book I have portrayed the Emoter as a bit of a crazy person, constantly driving self-destructive behaviors and having out-of-control desires. I've done this because it is sometimes true. If it wasn't, you wouldn't be struggling with whatever it is that motivated you to pick up this book. The Emoter can be a problem child.

The great news about the Emoter is that it always wants to feel *good*. We all want to be happy, feel fulfilled, and be content. Feeling like you have enough has everything to do with how you define what it takes for you to have those experiences. If you have a belief system that says you have to have a long list of certain things in order to be happy and you don't have those things, then you don't have enough.

You've discovered clarity about the experience of life you want; you've got your Thinker large and in charge; now I want you to challenge yourself deeply about what you have decided has to be in place for you to be happy. Make a conscious, self-driven choice about how much is enough.

This can be an amazingly freeing experience. I'll bet almost everyone reading this book has decided, at some point, that there is something you need to be happy that you don't have.

> **If you can find something that you thought you needed in order to please your Emoter, and it isn't necessary, the job just got easier.**

This is about making it easier to create a Willing Emoter. A smaller house, less stuff in the house, a cheaper car, the body you currently have, the job, spouse, kids or pets you currently have, etc. What do you have in your life that you see as not being good enough? If you look at it through the eyes of an Active Thinker, and with the clarity of your desired experience, you might just find that it is more than good enough.

Put Experiential Motivation to Work

The most effective way to get your Emoter on board with any new behavior is to find a way to couple it with an experience the Emoter enjoys or even craves. You do this by finding an experience the Emoter enjoys, within the activity you need to do. When you do, you are directly creating the experience you want, which is BE – DO – HAVE. You are in control because you are the source of the experience. Even if you don't get the outcome you might be after, you can still benefit from the experience of the action along the way. In short, use your desired experience as the motivator.

For example, many people have used this approach to enjoy exercise when they didn't previously. They got a workout buddy, signed up for dance classes or started golfing without renting the cart. They found a way to connect something they enjoy to the behavior they needed to do.

Jim uses this method to help him exercise. He knows that if his wife, Brenda joins him on his morning speed walk, his Emoter enjoys the connection. He also has this thing where after his walk he does a number of sit-ups and pushups that match his current age. His Emoter isn't thrilled with doing these actions, but something about feeling like he can do one more each year and being able to do that *really big* number, charges his Emoter. His Emoter enjoys the experience more than the action.

Jim's experience of exercise is feeling young and being connected to his wife. The Emotivators for him are accomplishment, challenge, and connection.

How can you use your desired experience, or your Emotivators, to fuel your Emoter during the behaviors you need to do?

Learn Something New

There are two benefits to new information. First, the Robot can't do it; the Robot tends to block out new information, so learning is done by the Thinker. By default, you are going around the Robot and the Thinker has to be awake in order to learn something new. Second, the Emoter likes to learn, at least when it is something you are interested in. Since motivation is really about pleasing the Emoter, your Emoter will be interested in any new learning that helps to create your desired experience.

So read a book, take a class, or talk with someone who is good at what you want to be good at. Just make sure your Active Thinker is choosing what you are going to learn. The Passive Thinker, when guided by the Emoter, is much more likely to grab a quick fix or look for a fad-like solution. If it seems too good to be true, it is. The real answers don't work overnight.

Other Tools for Motivating the Emoter

Sometimes it is difficult to find a way to use your desired purpose, or Emotivators, to help you enjoy an activity you need to do. If this is the case, you still have to find a way to get the Emoter on board and willing or it will always be a struggle. The following are some methods for doing that when your desired experience, or Emotivators, don't do the trick.

The Carrot

As I mentioned earlier, traveling is not my favorite part of my career but my Emoter doesn't rebel when I have to fly. It's an activity my Emoter is willing to do and it takes no will power to get myself to do it. I have found ways to make flying less miserable with movies, books, etc. But the main reason my Emoter is willing to do this behavior, is that it serves my Emotivators. My Emotivators don't show up during the event but it's what I have to do to get to the part where I do experience them. Traveling is a means to an end.

The carrot method of motivation is certainly not new, and I'm sure you've tried to use it many times without success. It's the main method companies use to motivate employees with rewards like raises, bonuses or promotions, often with disappointing results.

Most carrot-based motivation fails because we use a DO or a HAVE as the carrot, and it doesn't work long-term. Back to the work example: I frequently tell my clients that there is no such thing as a bonus. When someone gets a bonus, they are happy. Then, next year they think, "Where's my bonus?" It quickly turns into an expectation and the motivation wears off.

If the BE (an experience) is the carrot, it is much more effective.

You already use carrot-based motivation with great success, probably unconsciously. Look at all the things you do on a regular basis that your Emoter is okay with. Do you really love to brush your teeth, shower for work or take out the trash? Your Emoter has simply resigned itself to the fact that this is the way it is. There is no Emoter rebellion because you want the outcome enough to make it worth doing. As a result, the behavior long ago made it into your Robot, because you had a Willing Emoter.

You don't have to enjoy every action you take in life. Carrot-based motivation is when you use the outcome from the action to motivate you, not the action itself. When you use the BE or the experience of life as the carrot, it works better than using the DO or the HAVE. Carrot-based motivation does work, but only short term and in small doses. Most of your motivation needs to come from actions where you feel your desired experience or Emotivators while you are engaged in the behavior, not after it.

The Stick

Being motivated by fear is not an altogether bad thing. Fear often results in adverse effects in our lives, but only when we allow the Emoter to take over and keep the Thinker Passive. From the Emoter chapter:

> **When Active, we can ignore perceived threats that are not really dangerous and pay attention to, and be motivated by, real dangers.**

With a clear experience as a motivator coupled with an Active Thinker, the things you want to avoid or prevent can work to drive the Emoter in a positive direction. You should be afraid of being physically unhealthy, deeply in debt, stressed out of your mind, missing out on your children growing up, drifting away from your spouse, spending your days in a job you hate, etc. The only way these things would *not* motivate you is if you tuned them out.

Sometimes, reminding your Emoter of the negative consequences is necessary and effective. You just have to make sure they are not the only, or main motivators. You can use your fears, or the stick, as a wakeup call, and then focus on the good that you want to create, rather than the bad you want to avoid.

Replacement

Replacement is what the addiction field has been teaching for years as the way to break habits. It is the same method recommended by Charles Duhigg in *The Power of Habit – Why We Do What We Do in Life and Business*, that I mentioned in the Thinker chapter.

Replacement involves finding the emotional reward you achieve by performing an action you want to stop and finding a different, less destructive way to get your reward. In other words, find a better way to make the Emoter happy.

Take a look at the behaviors you are trying to stop or replace, and look for the payoff you get from the behavior.

Some examples:

- Shopping could really be about stress relief, time alone, time out of the house or building self-worth.

- Excessive worrying could be about feeling you are doing something without actually have to do something, or maybe getting to avoid a step you don't want to take.

- The payoff from having a crazy busy and stressful life could be about feeling valuable and important, or it could be a distraction from having to face a life you are not content with.

- Some people have found that being overweight is actually a protection from unwanted attention.

- When I worked in an office, the 3pm trip to the vending machine was really about taking a break and hanging out with friends.

- There are people who have affairs because they crave variety or because they love the challenge of seduction. There are better ways to experience variety and challenge.
- In my case, being broke was something I used as a motivator to get working. When things were going well, I didn't work as hard, but when money was tight, I was intensely focused.

What is your emotional reward? Underneath all unhealthy behavior lies an Emoter benefit. When you meet that desire in a different way, it will be much easier to stop the destructive action.

Willing Emoter Summary

Honor the Emoter
- We are conditioned to reject, avoid or suppress our emotions, often even when we feel good.
- The most crucial lesson to learn about creating a willing Emoter is to acknowledge that it exists, and to honor whatever the Emoter is feeling, good or bad.

How Much is Enough?
- What have you decided your Emoter needs in order to be happy? If you don't experience that happiness, you won't feel like you have enough. Make sure you truly need everything on your list.

- Challenge your thinking on how much is enough for you.

Put Your Emotivators to Work

- Find a way to connect the experience that motivates you to the actions you need to do.

The Carrot

- A carrot is an external motivator for the action you need to take. It is better when you are motivated by the action itself but sometimes that's just not possible.
- The most effective carrot is the promise of achieving your desired experience as a result of the activity you are engaged in.

The Stick

- There are things in life you should be afraid of. The Active Thinker can put these realities on the screen and use them to motivate the Emoter.
- While effective as a wakeup call, in the long run it is better to be motivated to move toward what you want, not away from what you don't want.

Learn Something New

- By default, new information is not currently in your Robot. Therefore, taking in new learning will change your perceptions and consequently, your emotional response.
- The Emoter likes to learn when learning serves the experience it wants. You feel more powerful, intelligent, and in control when you learn and because

the Emoter likes those feelings, it becomes more willing.

<u>Replacement</u>
- This is about finding the emotional reward you get by doing an undesirable action and finding a different, less destructive way to get your reward.

Support

Years ago, Jim was told by a former boss named Randy Revell, that the top thing he could do to become more successful was to surround himself with strong support. Jim said if he couldn't do it on his own, it didn't need to be done. Randy replied, "And that is your Achilles' heel." The programming of Jim's Robot, in regards to support, is not uncommon. The United States is an individualistic culture. Our values are self-sufficiency, self-reliance, and independence. We tend to regard needing support as a weakness. We feel we should be able to do it on our own.

Randy showed Jim some research done on Peak Performers – people at the top of their chosen field. They were asked why they were the best. The list had many similar answers, but there were only two in common on every list. One – they were clear on what they wanted (experientially motivated), which didn't surprise the researchers. But the second one did – they all talked about the value of support. They talked about the one coach who wouldn't let them slide, a parent who supported them when they wanted to quit, the boss who encouraged them to continue even after failure, or the friend who stood by them when others abandoned them.

Randy offered Jim the support that successfully helped him change his Robot. He now has a very strong belief that:

New Behavior Unsupported Becomes Extinct

The main function of support is to get and keep your Thinker Active. The well-worn grooves in your brain are easy to slip back into and without some kind of external help, it's unlikely you'll make it in the long run.

Support is important for a number of reasons:

- Remember the Active Thinker's job is to hold the present in one hand and the future in the other. Your desired experience of life is the glue that holds them together. The Thinker has to keep the hands together until the glue dries; you can think of support as a piece of rope tied around your hands to help you hold them in place long enough.

- Our brains tend to buy our own B.S. Let's say I'm on a diet, and there's a chocolate cake in front of me. My Emoter says, "I think cake is on my diet. It has eggs in it and that's protein." My Passive Thinker says, "If you say so." In a support system, we interrogate our own reality by running our thoughts through the contexts of others. A good support person would say, "I'm pretty sure cake is not on your diet." It's like outsourcing the Active Thinker role.

- We often keep our word with others more than we do with ourselves. Strange if you think about it, but true.

- You greatly increase the possibility that you will do what you say you are going to do if you set up a strong structure, and a deadline for getting the project done.

- Your brain loves patterns, which means patterns are hard to break. In a support structure, you tend to stay with new behavior long enough to break the pattern. On your own, not so much.

- Facing your fears is easier when you confront them with friends.

- A good support structure can snap you out of Passive and into Active Thinker. We all need a good wake-up call now and then.

- Active Thinkers like to hang out with Active Thinkers. Passive Thinkers like to hang out with Passive Thinkers. Who have you surrounded yourself with?

Rule #6 of the Internal Game is *Build a Good Team.* What does your team look like?

Time

Over the years, Oprah has been very open about her weight struggles, going through the same roller coaster gain/loss cycle that many others experience. One day, I was reading an article about a show she had recently done (when her show was still on the air). She had gained a bunch of weight and had her trainer on as a guest. She said something like, "I'm so frustrated and disappointed. How can I be here again? I know so much about the topic and have so much support; I thought I had it figured out. I thought I had it." Her trainer said, "That's the problem; you thought you had it so you stopped paying attention to it." What he was saying, was that she had turned the behavior back over to the Robot before it was ready.

How long does it take create a new habit? How long does it take to change the Robot? When I ask audiences this, people usually say twenty-one days, or something close to that number. Complete non-sense. There is no science to back up that old wives' tale. Oprah had lost the weight and kept it off much longer than twenty-one days. The real answer is – it depends. It depends on your Robot and how deeply ingrained the programming is that you are trying to overwrite.

Yes, this is a frustrating answer. I would love to give you a concrete number that your Emoter can work with. But the reality is that the time it takes can't be boiled down to something as simple as that.

You have to go into this change with a realistic expectation or it will never work. At the same time, if the expectation of time feels completely overwhelming, you'll have a very hard time getting the Emoter to be willing. So here are two rough guidelines for setting your time expectation.

Note the Small Victories

Rule #5 is *Life Happens Gradually, Then Suddenly*. One of the clearest areas where this rule applies is in the time it takes to change the Robot. The Emoter wants the sudden change – right now, which often actually short circuits your efforts to change. The key to using this rule is to learn how to pay attention to the gradual while it is happening. Often, the gradual happens in such small increments that your Passive Thinker can easily ignore or overlook them. One of the main jobs of the Active Thinker is to stay in touch with present reality and if you do this, you will be more aware of the gradual changes. With a good Active Thinker in charge, the small victories that don't feel like enough by themselves, can keep the Emoter willing to keep moving because you see your progress in the big picture and feel more and more of the experience that is driving you.

Overestimate Time

This second guideline suggests that you take whatever number you come up with for time expectations and double it. Most people guess far too low. I was talking with someone the other day who was having difficulties in her marriage. She realized that she was dealing with a lifelong pattern; she has never really felt happy and tends to blames the person she's with. We talked about therapy and she said, "I've tried therapy several times and it has never worked." When I pressed her about how long she usually went to therapy, she said that she never made it longer than a few months. I asked her how long she thinks she would have to go to make a difference, and she said probably a *whole year*, as if that was an eternity. I encouraged her to set her sights on at least two.

As for Oprah, I think there might be some areas of our lives that we will continually have to manage using the Active Thinker. What she was really saying to her trainer was, "I turned off my Thinker and gave control over to the Robot."

There may be small pieces of eating or exercise that are now automatic for her and she doesn't have to pay attention to them, but it is likely that she will always have to remain at least partially conscious of this area. Don't let this discourage you. While the area you want to change might be like Oprah's, and you will always have to keep an Active Thinker monitoring it, it does get easier. Staying on top of it is significantly easier than climbing the mountain to get to the top. Just give yourself the time to get there.

Robot Reprogramming Summary

The short summary of this chapter goes like this:

- **Motivation** – What's the experience you want to create?
- **Active Thinker** – What is present reality and what future are you going to create?
- **Willing Emoter** – How much resistance do you have to the changes and how are you going to keep your Emoter on board?
- **Support** – What kind of support do you need?
- **Time** – How much time will this take?

These are the five components you need to satisfy, and to imbed new programming into your Robot. A much more detailed approach follows. You can use this as a worksheet to put a plan in place for yourself. Go to the website to download an electronic version:

www.NeverEnoughNation.com

Robot Reprogramming Worksheet

Motivation

<u>Experiential Motivation</u>
- WHY do you want this change? What is the experience of life you are going to create?

- **Emotivators**

    o **Safety** – Do you feel safe? If not, how so and why?

    o **Pleasure** – How can you consciously give your Emoter positive experiences through your senses?

    For each of the following, choose the word or words that you feel most captures your experience of each need.

    o **Acceptance** – The experience of being valued and valuable. Everyone needs to feel love, and acceptance is the root experience of love. Self-Acceptance trumps acceptance from others.
    Similar experiences: Recognition, Being the Center of Attention, Being Impressive, Belonging, Acknowledgement, Being Seen/Noticed, Being the Best, Feeling Attractive.

    o **Independence** – The experience of being different from the tribe, being an individual, and believing you can survive on your own.

Similar experiences: Freedom, Autonomy, Uniqueness, Self-Determination, Being Special, Variety.

○ **Contribution** – The experience of adding value to others or the world.
Similar experiences: Nurturing, Adding Value to a Cause Greater than Yourself, Making a Difference, Purpose.

○ **Accomplishment** – The need to feel you can do something. In order to feel all is right with the world, your Emoter must have a sense that it can get something done.
Similar experiences: Mastery, Challenge, Achievement, Creativity, Order from Chaos, Organizing, Problem Solving.

○ **Knowledge** – The experience of having knowledge or the experience of acquiring it. Your Emoter likes to know that it knows things or can figure things out. Some are driven more by having the knowledge and others by the acquisition of knowledge.
Similar experiences: Discovery, Insight, Wisdom, Learning, Innovation, Problem Solving, Creativity.

Active Thinker

<u>Managing Your Screen</u>
- *Embrace Present Reality* – What is the present reality of your life? What are your results and what damaging behaviors are you using?
- *Be Right about the Right Things* – What have you been being right about to your own detriment?
- *Own the Game* – How have you allowed yourself to feel like a victim?

<u>Track the Future</u>
- What is your plan for having your desired experience show up?
- Do you need some goals?

<u>Get Out of Your Comfort Zone</u>
- How will you challenge your comfort zone?

<u>Build a Stronger Thinker</u>
- How will you keep yourself sharp?

Willing Emoter Summary

<u>Honor the Emoter</u>
- What are your feelings about your plan and the path forward? Good, bad or otherwise, honor and acknowledge that those feelings exist.

<u>How Much is Enough?</u>
- What have you decided you need that you can challenge and let go of?

Put Experiential Motivation to Work
- Find a way to connect your desired experience to the actions you need to do.

The Carrot
- What carrots can you use to help keep the Emoter willing?

The Stick
- What are some realities you have been avoiding that you need to handle?

Learn Something New
- What can you learn about this area of your life?

Replacement
- Considering the damaging behaviors you have been using, what is the emotional payoff you've been getting from them?
- How are you going to get those payoffs in more effective ways?

Support
- What types of changes do you need to make to your environment or the structure of your life that will support you in actualizing your desired experience?

Time

- How much time do you think it will take to make the changes you desire a permanent part of your Robot?
- What are some small victories that you can look for as evidence of the gradual, then sudden changes?

9

Success Stories

In the Introduction, I said that for most of the book, we would talk about health, wealth, and stress together, because what we cover reaches beneath each of them, to what they all have in common. Now, we are going to explore each of them individually.

I believe that if you look at most people who have been successful at creating long-term change, you'll discover that they found a way to address the five components of the Robot Reprogramming Formula: an intrinsic and experiential motivation that drives an Active Thinker + Willing Emoter + Support + Time.

To help illustrate this, we're going to look at three case studies of real people who have created real change, and we'll examine how they went about it. In other words, let's take a look at the formula in action. I'll start each section with some thoughts about the topic itself, as well as some resources or suggestions I've found valuable; then I'll tell you a bit about each person's story, explaining how they addressed the five components of the Robot Reprogramming Formula. Keep in mind that these people didn't have the worksheet to follow when they changed. In fact, I didn't even show it to them when I interviewed them. I just asked them to tell me how they did it; their answers filled in the blanks. This helped prove to me that these are the elements that are needed to create change.

You have the benefit of the Robot Reprogramming Worksheet, which hopefully will make your path easier. Your challenge is to chart your own course, using the worksheet and drawing inspiration from these examples of others who succeeded.

Managing Your Health

Which of the three areas is the most difficult to manage? The answer is, whichever one is most challenging for you. But of the three, I believe physical health is the area with the greatest amount of negative societal pressures. It's undesirable to be deeply in debt but it's hard to know that about someone just by looking at them. In some ways, being stressed is almost expected and not even seen as a negative. But being over-weight brings quick and nearly universal negative judgments. Of the three, I believe it is the one that strikes most deeply at the core of self-acceptance, and as such, can be the most painful.

If this is the area that is most challenging for you, I want to start by reminding you about the "Honor the Emoter" section we covered in the last chapter. Shame and self-loathing are not effective motivators. While I'm not asking you to ignore or dismiss feelings of displeasure with your current situation, I don't want you to be motivated by them alone. What I want you to do is strive for and create the experience of life you desire. In other words, this is not about getting rid of what's wrong with you or about making you a better, more acceptable person.

We've talked at length about the many temptations that surround you – more than ever before in history. The largest of these temptations is food. If you eat what you are most exposed to, you will be unhealthy. It's a shame but what is, is. Liking it or not liking it won't change it. The bottom line is that our food supply is making us a very sick and unhealthy nation.

The best resource I've found on the subject is the New York Times bestseller, *It Starts with Food: Discover the Whole30 and Change Your Life in Unexpected Ways* by Dallas and Melissa Hartwig. It explains the science and biology of food in a clear and easy to follow way. Here's a question for you: if you had to choose, would you rather have physical health or financial health? I'm guessing you said physical. Now ask yourself, which one do you know the most about and spend the most time tracking and managing? Most would say financial. If this is true for you, I strongly encourage you to learn more about and pay closer attention to your physical health.

The Story of Trisha

"I went on my first diet when I was six years old," Trisha said. "My Grandmother told me she'd buy me two new outfits if I lost weight. I was never obese but I was always chunky. I was the fat kid everyone made fun of."

Trisha's story is an impressive one. Currently a single mother, she struggled with her weight throughout her childhood. Today, she is at her ideal weight and has kept it there for more than twelve years. Trisha met Randy, her now ex-husband, in 1995 when she was twenty-two years old. At the time, she weighed about one hundred and eighty pounds at five-feet, ten-inches. By 1998, after being with Randy for three years, her weight had increased to two hundred and thirty-five pounds. "I gained it so slowly that I didn't notice," Trisha said. Then in one year, she lost eighty-five pounds. As I tell the rest of this story, I'll break down what she told me into the five variables of the Robot Reprogramming Formula.

Motivation

"In January 1999, I was looking at holiday pictures and I saw how much bigger I was than everyone else. I tore up all the pictures." This was Trisha's bottoming out moment. Many people don't start working on change until they hit some kind of crisis; this was hers. Sometimes it takes a tipping point like this to wake you up to the true experience of life that you are having every day.

Her success didn't come from an external focus on body image. She certainly tracked her progress, but she was motivated by how she felt and how she wanted to feel, not just by how she looked.

"After the first three months, I had lost forty pounds. I remember crying when the scale showed I weighed less than two hundred pounds again. I'm never going back. I don't want to be fat and frumpy. I don't want to be the fat chick – I've been that girl." Talking to her, you can feel her Emoter radiating the happiness she experiences in her life today.

"I feel so much lighter, physically and emotionally. It was harder just to move, put clothes on, and enjoy life. I really didn't feel good about myself then." Trisha was motivated by her experience of life, not just by her circumstances.

Active Thinker

The challenge to keeping the Thinker Active is to hold the present in your left hand, hold the future in the right, have a plan for bringing them together, and then hold both tightly until they are one. The clarity of how she wanted to BE combined with a sure vision of the future, gave her the motivation she needed.

During Trisha's weight loss period, her Thinker came up with a plan to create that future. She got a Cooking Light book that she used to make her dinners. She came home from work every day, exercised for forty-five minutes using a workout video, and then cooked a healthy meal using recipes from the book. She packed her lunches and limited alcohol intake. As she got stronger, she added heavier weights to her routine and used more challenging videos. She didn't go to the gym because she was too embarrassed about her body. In short, she ate right and exercised. It sounds simple but I know that it can be difficult. She didn't use a fad diet or go to crazy extremes. According to Trisha, "You can't go on a strict diet. At least I can't – it just doesn't work."

That was the plan her Thinker put together. I asked her how she stays focused now and how she has done it for so long. She told me about one of the best strategies I've heard for *Embracing Present Reality*, Rule #1. She said, "I'm very aware of what I eat now. I make smaller adjustments, plus or minus five pounds. I stopped weighing myself last year. My clothes are a size ten and I can tell what I weigh by how tight or loose they feel. If they feel tight, I put on my skinniest jeans and keep wearing them until they fit right."

Most people, when their clothes start to get tight, go to larger clothes or their "fat" jeans. Trisha has a great strategy in place for keeping the present firmly in her left hand. Being fully aware and awake to what is currently real is a major piece of an Active Thinker's job. While the Robot is changing, the Thinker has to remain aware of both the present and the future; because there is a gap between them, it takes much more work. Once the present becomes the desired image of the future, the Thinker just needs to monitor the present to make sure it remains consistent. Trisha's Thinker was fully engaged during her weight loss, and has consistently performed its monitoring role ever since.

Willing Emoter

"During the weight loss, I started therapy. I figured out that I was eating to suppress emotion. I was self-medicating." Trisha dug in during this process and uncovered some repressed memories of abuse from her childhood. The abuse was a major discovery, as was the way she applied the concept of "replacement" that we discussed in the last chapter under Willing Emoter. Destructive behaviors give you some kind of Emoter benefit or you wouldn't do them. In Trisha's case, eating was suppressing emotions she didn't know how to deal with.

"I can still feel urges to eat junk when I'm stressed. Now I use exercise to reduce stress but I still eat junk sometimes." Today, Trisha goes to the gym four times a week while being a single mom, working a full time job, going to school, and maintaining a relationship.

Trisha was motivated to create a different way of being; she was moved to get away from a result she didn't want and along the way, found a different way to satisfy what the Emoter was getting from over-eating and being over-weight. Keeping the Emoter willing while giving the Robot the time needed to change often takes a combination of strategies.

Support

"Randy was a big support for me. He lost about twenty-five pounds during that time. Sometimes, when I didn't want to exercise, he would do it with me. I dedicated my life to it for six months." Trisha had the benefit of being kid-free at the time and having a significant other who was willing to do the work with her: both very helpful. She also got rid of all the junk food in the house.

"I went to my doctor and begged for pills. He was reluctant to give them to me but they were a big help. He checked out all my vital statistics first and was blown away when I came back three months later, forty pounds lighter." She used medication to help her but did not rely on it to do all the work.

Over the last twelve years, Trisha has maintained an active social life, going to bars, pool parties, boating, etc. She credits these situations, where she is very aware of what she is wearing and how she looks, with playing a major supporting role in helping her keep the weight off. Who you surround yourself with plays a big role in your results.

It is very difficult to make lasting change on our own. You will be hard-pressed to find someone who has been successful, who didn't make changes in their environment and support system.

Time

Trisha doesn't describe this area of her life as done. "It's something I always have to pay attention to," she says, "But it's much easier today." It may well be that Trisha's Robot will never be able to run her physical health completely on auto pilot. It has been changed and as a result, even in auto pilot mode her Emoter is driven to do some healthy things like exercising. As mentioned earlier though, there is a big difference between the work it takes to get on top of an area and the work it takes to stay there. It took Trisha a good two to three years to climb to the top and switch over to maintenance mode. And she's stayed on top for about ten years now.

Managing Your Wealth

If the food we are exposed to is the biggest of the temptations we face, money is a close second. In the last section, I encouraged you to learn more about food and nutrition and I'll do the same with money. Check out *Pocket Your Dollars: 5 Attitude Changes That Will Help You Pay Down Debt, Avoid Financial Stress, and Keep More of What You Make,* by Carrie Rocha, or the books you'll hear about in the following story.

Most of us, including me, received little or no education about money management while we were growing up. I learned how to manage a checkbook from the woman at the bank where I opened my first account. The bank was just off my college campus, and she was so accustomed to clueless freshmen coming in that she had developed her own little miniature course. It wasn't enough.

Money is a taboo topic in America, just like weight. You're just not supposed to talk about them. The lack of open, honest dialogue or even confrontation, is a major flaw in our social structure. I believe that we need to bring this topic out into the open and make it standard education in our schools. The good news is that some states are doing this, but not many. I also think that organizations should provide education to employees; some do.

Most people would rather be healthy than wealthy, but fortunately, you don't have to choose between the two; you can have both. But how do you define wealthy? It means very different things to different people. The creeping ideals and expectations of the American Dream have greatly distorted how people answer that question. My challenge to you is to figure out how you define wealthy. How much is enough for you, and how have you chained your experience of life to this area?

The Story of Matthew

Matthew, who happens to be bald, owns and operates a hair salon on the north side of Seattle (James Alan Salon & Spa for those in the area; we recommend it.) The salon has about thirty employees, little debt, and has been ranked one of the best places to work in Washington State. It has an employee turnover well below the industry average, a client retention rate above the industry average, shows respectable profits, and is valued between $500 and $750 thousand. Matthew has no personal debt. In addition to the Salon, he owns a condo and has $250 thousand in retirement savings. He's single and recently celebrated his fiftieth birthday. But he hasn't always enjoyed such financial stability.

As a child, he was exposed to constant financial woes. He remembers when the repo people came and took the family's television and his mom's sewing machine. They received food stamps and usually made use of the free lunch program at school. Matthew started working as a babysitter at age eleven so that he could buy clothes; he has been working ever since. But even with a strong and early work ethic, he followed his parents' example, spending everything he made as soon as, or even sooner than, he made it.

Fast forward to 1993. Matthew is in a relationship and has $35 thousand in credit card debt. He's making car payments and has recently purchased a newly constructed house for about $250 thousand. He is also making payments and keeping up with maintenance costs on a cabin in the mountains, and he has no real savings. The combined family income is between $80 and $90 thousand.

He said, "One of the dumbest things I've ever done with money is cashing in my 401k when I left my job. It had fifteen hundred dollars in it. I paid five hundred dollars in taxes and penalties and spent the remaining one thousand on carpeting for my house. If I had money, I spent it."

While Matthew's situation was certainly not good, there are stories that are much worse. I chose his story because it's not rags to riches – it's more broke to doing very well. At the worst of his financial woes, his situation was actually very close to that of the average American. I believe his path is one that most people will be able to relate to. Let's see how he did it.

Motivation

Matthew's was not a bottoming-out experience. His situation was not good but he was not in crisis. He made a considerable investment in his financial education without a specific crisis driving him. Instead, he was motivated by his desire to learn and improve himself.

His motivation to change his experience of wealth was aroused while talking with a support person he met during a series of courses called *The Excellence Series*, by Context

International. The company's personal and professional growth programs encourage people to look at their lives while teaching skills like motivation, relationship building, and stepping out of your comfort zone. He had been involved in these courses for a number of months before having this pivotal conversation.

"I was talking with a friend and support person, and he told me I should sell our cabin. I said, no, it's an investment! I was angry at the suggestion. He asked how much we pay on it, and I said four hundred and fifty a month. He asked how often we go there and I hesitantly said, about twice a year. He did the math, and said five thousand four hundred dollars would pay for a heck of a bed and breakfast trip twice a year. This was a real wake-up call for me. That was my "Ah Ha" moment."

Not only did that conversation wake him up to the errors in his thinking about money, it also helped connect him to a deep and compelling experiential motivation. He believed that because he wasn't destitute like he was during his childhood, he was doing well. But his experience of life was based on a fantasy. This often happens for people in the area of wealth; they feel okay and are having a good experience of life, even when it's not based in reality. If you live as though you have something you don't, it can make you feel good. But when reality comes knocking, it can be an ugly visit. Fortunately for Matthew, he broke out of his fantasy world and created a genuine experience of wealth rather than the artificial one he was inhabiting.

In other words, his wakeup call didn't help him see the experience of life he was missing, it helped him see that his experience of life was a lie. He felt like he had wealth and lived like he had wealth, but he didn't. He was motivated to create the experience of life he thought he had until he got in touch with reality.

Active Thinker

"There were two books that really influenced me," Matthew said. *"The Wealthy Barber* and *Your Money or Your Life.* In the latter, there is an exercise that asks you to add up all the money you've ever made including the lawn mowing, babysitting, etc. and then figure out your true hourly rate for what you currently make. Both really surprised me and gave me a new way of looking at spending money."

This exercise is a great example of all three rules that show up while working to "Manage Your Screen." Adding up all the money he had ever made was a cold, hard way for Matthew to *Embrace Present Reality,* Rule #1. When he compared the money he had made to the money he had at the time, he was shocked to see how little he had held onto. That kicked his Thinker into Active mode and got his Emoter's attention.

The second exercise was to figure out his real hourly rate. For example, let's say someone makes $45 thousand per year. Let's assume forty-five hours per week, two weeks' vacation per year, add in another ten days for holidays and sick leave, and a net tax rate of twenty percent after deductions. That comes out to an hourly rate of just under seventeen dollars. Now calculate commuting time, transportation costs, work clothes, job education, and any other job related expenses, and add that to your work costs. Now your hourly rate may look more like thirteen dollars. Next, convert everything you buy into hours. Do you buy a four-dollar latte at Starbucks every morning? That will cost you about six hours of work each month. This is where Rule

#2 comes in – *Be Right About the Right Things*. It's easy to think, "Sure, I can afford a latte. I deserve it," and feel right about that. But when you put the true cost of that latte on the screen for your Emoter – six hours of your life, it's no longer a question of, "Can you afford it?" Now it's a choice of what is most important to you. A new car for $22 thousand would cost one thousand, six hundred and ninety-two hours or just over thirty-seven weeks, not including tax or interest if you finance it. That's seventy-two percent of an entire year's work for a car. It's hard to feel "right" about being able to afford that.

Both these methods helped Matthew with Rule #3 – *Own the Game*. He was making normal, mainstream choices: buy a house, get a car, acquire some credit cards – all standard things to do. Unfortunately, going with the flow of today's society will wreck your health and wealth and raise your stress levels. Matthew wasn't in charge of his game; the societal forces around him were.

For Matthew, this was not just an exercise in logic. This was about putting information in front of his Emoter so that change could happen without relying on will power. The Emoter feels very differently about that latte and everything else you buy when you see how much of your life's energy it will cost you. Your motivation changes without the Thinker having to overpower the Emoter.

Willing Emoter

The main method Matthew used to keep his Emoter on board was his understanding of what drives his Emoter. He knew that three of his Emotivators were accomplishment, challenge, and creativity. He was able to intentionally and consciously create these experiences while changing his habits.

"I did a budget on a spreadsheet. There was a column for each area. If there was no money in the column, we couldn't spend it. I got really energized by it." While he was telling me the story, I could hear his excitement and enthusiasm. Budgeting was a game Matthew's Emoter was engrossed in, because his experience of life in the moment was accomplishment, challenge, and creativity. The side effect was better financial health. BE – DO – HAVE. "I loved paying off a credit card, then taking that money and making bigger payments on the next card," Matthew said. He had developed a very effective way to keep his Emoter not only willing, but charged and engaged in the new behavior.

Support

Matthew had a ton of support in place to help him create and maintain his new habits. He stayed involved in the series of courses I mentioned earlier. In one of the courses he took, he became part of a support group that stayed together for ten years. He read books that helped him understand how money works, and then formed a *Your Money or Your Life* group at his office. The group went through the workbook version of the book for six months. He not only put the group together, but he also led it.

After taking a look at all the support he had in place, Matthew said, "I hadn't thought about how much support I had. I don't have that in place with my physical health, which is probably why I still struggle there." Matthew is actually in good shape. His version of struggling is being five to ten pounds overweight, and usually not even that. But notice how much more work that area of his life feels like to his Emoter because he has not yet applied the winning formula.

Time

I asked Matthew about the time it took to make these changes. He said, "It's more unconscious now but I had to stay really conscious for the first four to six years. Now it's intuitive." "Now" is about ten years later. Real change is not a quick fix.

<u>Manage Your Stress</u>

Of the three areas: money, food, and stress, stress has been by far the most difficult for finding a good success story. As a nation, we recognize that being broke and/or overweight is bad, but stressed – that's another story. In the work place, many people automatically start conversations with, "I know you're busy, but..." We don't approach people and say, "I know you're over-weight, but..." We just assume that anyone we think highly of must be busy and stressed out. If you are not stressed, you must be lazy, a deadbeat, unemployed or otherwise have something wrong with you. In our culture, we not only think it is okay to live a high-stress lifestyle, we expect it.

Given the cultural acceptance, and even expectation of being stressed, I want to start this section by challenging you to *Own Your Game*, Rule #3. Are you a victim of social pressure in this area?

The story you are about to hear is that of the second person I interviewed for this section. The first one had a great story. She started with, "I had the full catastrophe." Then went on to talk about how she went from being an overworked, over-stressed, successful member of the corporate rat race to working four hours a day from home and living a life of experiential abundance. But because she is single and her kids are grown, people easily dismissed her example. From the beta-readers, I heard things like, "Well sure, if I didn't have to deal with kids or a spouse and could get by on four hours of work a day, my life would be a breeze too." I didn't want to give anyone that easy an out, so I found a different example.

My challenge to you is, instead of looking at the following example and finding problems or circumstances you have that she doesn't, own your game. If you're stressed, don't blame it on your circumstances. Either change your circumstances, or change the way you look at your life, or both.

I also could have used Matthew from the wealth example as a success story about stress, because he is the busiest person I know but he doesn't feel stressed or even busy. I need a nap just listening to him tell me about his schedule. But it works for him. In fact, he loves it.

This brings us to the question, "What is stress?" At the deepest and most basic level, stress is fear. Matthew is not stressed because he has designed and crafted a life that allows him to feel safe WHILE his Emoter has a positive experience. His basic safety needs are met and he feels certain that his life will give him the BE his Emoter wants.

The biggest driver of stress in the American culture is the DO – HAVE – BE approach. It does create some happiness, which is why most people would say their life is okay or even a little better than okay. But the amount of work you have to put into that machine to get a little trickle of BE out the other side is stressful. The fear comes from feeling that you are not doing it right, or that it won't keep working.

That stress often drives the *more* approach and the temptations behind the Never Enough Mindset.

The Story of Michelle

Michelle is a thirty-seven year old single mother of two children, eight and ten years old. She works as a mid-level manager at a technology company, currently leading a team of five, and has led teams of five to twenty in the past. She has been with her current employer since 1997 but took four years off when she had her children. She works forty to forty-five hours a week, thirty of those in the office, and the rest at home or remotely. Michelle is very successful in her career and has a great reputation; she consistently receives positive reviews and is being given ever-increasing responsibilities as she rises through the ranks in a very competitive and workaholic culture. She has a boyfriend, exercises five days a week, and regularly volunteers at her kids' school. Those are the circumstances of her life, but what is more important is her experience of life. She's happy and has a low level of stress, but that wasn't always true. Let's look at how she got there.

Motivation

"For me, stress happens when I'm not following my own priorities," Michelle said. "I think the driver behind many people's stress is guilt. They have a big project to do at work, their family wants them home, and there is only one of them to go around. They are constantly trying to figure out how to manage all the competing demands on their time. Time is my most valuable resource. It is the one that I can't make more of and that I have to manage most carefully."

A major component of stress is time management. Michelle places a high value on her time because she knows it is the only place where experiences occur. If your time is used up with experiences you don't value, you won't have time to create the experiences you do value. Of the four years she took away from her career to have her children, she said, "I chose to walk away from what I felt would still be there four years later."

But when she went back to work as a mother and recent divorcee, she fell into the DO – HAVE – BE trap.

"I felt this tremendous need to prove myself, especially as a single mom. I put in a lot of hours at the office and at home, 8pm – 11pm every night. I needed to do it for a short period of time to get a major project off the ground. But it did not bring me personal fulfillment. My project was okay and my kids were alive, but I wanted more."

The "more" she was talking about was the quality of her experience of life. Her BE wasn't showing up. "I used to feel like I was racing every day – racing to beat the clock, to pick my kids up on time from their after school program, to get home, slam down some dinner, and then do homework, laundry, other basic essentials. Then it was time for the kids to go to bed. I had very little quality time with them. I felt like I was always running late. I was barely on time for meetings or for picking up my kids. I didn't want to be that kind of role model. I didn't want them to think, 'Sure, Mom has this great job but she's crazy. Mom doesn't take great care of herself. Mom doesn't nurture her social relationships.'"

This was where her motivation came from: the recognition that she was not having the experience of life she wanted. She decided, "I'm going to think a lot about what my priorities are, and I'm going to be really transparent about them with the people around me. They can like me or not, but I'm going to follow my priorities day in and day out, and that way, I'm not going to have a conflict about what I'm doing or more importantly, not doing. That will help me be relatively un-stressed."

Michelle is clear about her desired experience of life, and she works consistently and creatively to generate it on a daily basis. She understands that this applies to her physical health as well. "There is a big difference between losing weight to fit into a bikini this summer versus losing weight because you want to be a better person, serve as a better role model, and live a better life." Let's look at how she puts this experiential clarity into action.

Active Thinker

The present reality that Michelle held in her left hand was over-stressed, over-worked, and not experiencing quality time with her children. Next she needed to figure out the future she wanted to create and hold that in her right hand. "I made a list of non-negotiables in my head. I want to do a lot of things with my kids at school because I'll never get to do them again. I want to be there with them. I want to support their education. I want to be there in their classroom. I not only want to do the fun stuff at school, but also be a reading and math assistant once a month. By doing that, I'm supporting their goal, which is their education and for me, that's non-negotiable. I take time off work for almost every school activity. It's not one hundred percent non-negotiable because sometimes conflicts come up and I have to miss something, but most of the time, I'm there." She was clear about the future she wanted to create, both tangibly and intangibly. The next part was the plan for bringing the two together. Here's how she did it:

"I started cutting my hours three managers ago and I did it in the dark. I didn't say anything, I just started doing it. I figured that at the end of the year, I would know how I was doing with my job. I knew it would be good for my family but I didn't know what it would do for my career. At the end of the year, I got a great review and a promotion. So then I decided I can keep doing this and I don't have to keep being so squirrelly about it. I'm going to actually make a schedule and put it in my calendar. It's a standard, recurring meeting in my Outlook." The recurring meeting on her schedule shows her booked from 8am to 10am and from 4pm through the rest of the day. The schedule only shows space from 10am to 4pm, so if someone tries to schedule her for a meeting, that's when they have to do it.

Michelle said, "I just transitioned to a new and very well-regarded manager a couple of weeks ago. Four weeks ago, he recruited me for his team, so I figured, 'This is my best shot. I'm just going to put my cards on the table.' I told him, 'I have office hours from ten to four, and then I work the rest of my day from home, or remotely.' He said, 'I didn't know that but I do know that you get a crap ton done.'" She was unclear what unit of measure "crap ton" constituted, but those were his exact words.

"I've gone from 'this is an experiment' to 'I'm going to document this' to 'I'm going to talk about this.' I don't think smart people are going to say, 'Gosh, if your butt is not in your chair sixty hours a week, I don't think I can hire you for my team.' I think people are more likely to look at your results, especially if you are a decent and reasonable person while you are achieving those results. I know so many people who are overworked and unpleasant as a result. You can't get through a conversation without hearing them complain: 'Oh, I wish I could do that but I have meetings booked until 8pm.' Okay, I'm sorry, but one of those meetings can't be as important as something else. There must be something you can cut out of your day if your life is that messed up."

This is the part where you might think, "That would never work at my company or in my career." And you may be right. I don't know your situation. Please don't get fired and call me. Call Jim instead.

Actually, I think this would work at most companies. There are people who are still naïve enough to think that counting hours equals productivity but in most companies, if you make the case that even with shorter hours you are as productive or more so than your co-workers, this would work. Many organizations are providing flexible hours and placing more value on work-life balance. More companies are emulating, thinking of emulating or know they should be emulating this model. If yours is not, maybe you can lead them there, or you might have to make a choice about what is most important to you.

I digress. Michelle's plan followed Rule # 6 – *Life Happens Gradually, then Suddenly.* She didn't just walk in one day and give an ultimatum about working fewer hours. She put her plan in place, little by little, so much so that others didn't even notice. Her results spoke for themselves.

She also uses her Active Thinker to be creative and to problem solve. "I'm sure I said 'no' to people who would have rather heard me say 'yes,' but I tried to do a good job with the messaging. I would say, 'I'm sorry, I'm not available at that time. Let me know what the action items are that you need me to do after the meeting.' If it was someone I really wanted to work with, I would go so far as to message them later that night and say, 'Hey, while it's still fresh on your mind, is there anything that you need me to know from that meeting?' This is a pretty effective way of skipping a meeting; I just spent thirty seconds making it clear that I was willing to help and be part of the team, without sitting in an hour-long meeting. If people recognize that you are willing to work hard and be part of the team, they're going to forgive the small time-related issues along the way."

Another example she gave: if a meeting is crucial, she volunteers to schedule it. She looks like a go-getter for stepping up, and she controls the timing. "I want to participate and contribute, which often means showing up! So I try to set important meetings during my core hours," she said.

I asked if she felt any pressure from her company to work more hours. What I was really asking was, "How do you manage your screen?" If she constantly felt that she was under scrutiny or in the process of failing, her Emoter would be feeling major stress.

She said a couple of things: "If you want to do a lot of things, it's possible to be fully present for each one of those things, as long as you don't pack more into a given day than you can handle. There are things you can cut that people don't know you can cut, and that you just don't need in your life."

She also said, "The people I respect at work, many of whom are above me in the hierarchy, are not killing it on hours. Anyone can go in and work sixty hours. That's not a skill. Anyone can put their butt in a chair sixty hours a week. It's really what you do with your time, how you interact with other people, and the results of your work, not the time you spend."

What she's talking about here is how she "Managed her Screen" and Rule #2 – *Be Right About the Right Things.* One of the most common comments I hear from people who work insane hours is that they have no choice; it's the only way they can succeed. Michelle's company is notorious for its workaholic culture and she could have been "right" about that being the only way to win in that environment. Instead, she chose to believe that she could be successful by working fewer hours, and keeping that on her screen until it became a permanent part of her Robot.

<u>Exercise</u>

Exercise not only builds a stronger Thinker, it is also a fantastic stress reliever. Talking about exercise, Michelle said, "I put the kids on the bus and go to the gym five days a week. It really helps me clear my mind, and I find it enormously beneficial to my body. If I haven't moved my major muscle groups, by two or three in the afternoon I can get a little cranky. I feel that I'm better at work because I exercised in the morning, and I feel that almost every single day. I'm much more relaxed if I beat it out on the treadmill rather than arguing it out in a meeting. I feel we function better as human beings when we use our bodies in the way they were designed to be used."

Willing Emoter

In the Willing Emoter section of the last Chapter, one of the sections was "How Much is Enough?" This is not only one of the biggest questions of this entire book, it's the single biggest contributor to stress. It's ironic that trying to do too much can create the feeling of not enough. To get her stress under control, Michelle had to examine her definition of "enough."

"I won't take on projects that won't work. I was asked to be part of a project that had meetings scheduled from 5 to 6pm every day, so I passed on the project. Maybe that was stupid from the 'take every project to make your manager happy' point of view but it would have hurt me more in my overall experience of life."

When those kinds of conflicts come up, Michelle goes back to her priorities. She may feel an emotional pull from the project but she may also feel a bigger emotional pull in a different direction. If she did not have deep clarity about what is most important to her, her BE, it would be much harder to say "no."

"I do bend or flex on my schedule at times but there are limits. People say 'yes' to one little thing that leads to another and another, and the next thing they know they are working seventy hours a week, their spouse has left, and their kids don't know them."

"I feel this is a major problem today: husbands and wives are trying to do things to please each other but they are failing. I know a ton of people at the office who are working long days to get a promotion to please their wives. In reality, their wives are at home thinking, 'Dinner is cold, and you're a jerk.'"

Michelle knows how to work with her Emoter to keep from getting overly stressed. "At the end of the day, I use a 'Saving State,' which is a computer expression that means capture your thoughts so that you can make a clean exit from that moment and make a clean entry later. Driving away from the office and still thinking about the job doesn't work. I'd probably get in a car crash because I'm a very intense thinker.

I need to check out in order to walk out the door." Many people carry their work around in their heads everywhere they go. It's one of the reasons they have a hard time leaving at the end of the day. They can't turn off their work brain. Indeed, it's very hard to do if you don't have something else to put in front of the Emoter.

"At the end of the day, there is the question of, 'do I need to leave at four?' I don't *have* to get my kids by four-thirty. Every day I have to kick myself in the butt to get up and leave because I want to go play with my kids. That's a fun reason. I don't have to make a choice to do something that isn't fun. If I'm forty-five minutes away from finishing something, it can be really tempting to stay. Occasionally, I'll do that; maybe twenty percent of the time I'll stay late, and it's okay for me to do that one day a week. You can't build a structure so rigid that you can't move; that causes its own stress."

Support

"I do have a personal life. I do check in at work in the evening, but it's just a quick check-in. I have a boyfriend who gives me great emotional and intellectual support. We both have a strong sense of self, so after the kids go to bed we make the time we need for us as a couple and as individuals."

Michelle has intentionally created a relationship that supports her values and lifestyle, rather than one which requires her to frequently bend over backwards to support the relationship. "Someone once told me, you don't have time for a boyfriend unless he adds value to your life. I said, 'Wow, I cannot think of a human being in terms of value-added.' But at the same time, that person was probably not far off base. I don't have time for a dramatic relationship where I'm expected to cater to my partner's needs. I also don't have time for a man who is more like a third child. I found a strong guy who is like-minded in terms of values, who is super smart, and great at his job, and who wants me to be great at my job too. We give each other a lot of positive support and we have a high degree of mutual respect."

Michelle has also structured her life to support the things she wants to do. "It's important for me to not give myself any outs. When I get out of bed, I put my workout clothes on right way. If I decided to skip the gym, I would have to take them off and put on my work clothes, and that would feel really foolish. I have one less wardrobe change if I do it in the morning. If I don't do it in the morning, it doesn't get done. Putting myself first really only happens on the blank slate part of the day – and that's the morning. Later in the day, work, picking up the kids, and any number of other things get in the way. I know my weaknesses, so I put my gym clothes on right away; I have to either go to work looking very silly or get my body to the gym. I've programmed my days to meet the goals I want to achieve."

Time

The time it took for Michelle to make the change from typical corporate world hard worker living "the full catastrophe" to a highly successful, dedicated, and abundantly available mom in a healthy relationship spanned ten years. It took almost two years just to change her work hours. It wasn't quick but all things considered, very impressive.

The last thing Michelle told me was, "While chaperoning my son's class field trip last month, I had six of his classmates in the car and just listened to them while I drove. On that trip, I learned more about my son than by asking him about his day, every day since September.

"It's not about letting your career die on the vine. Every person can reclaim an hour or two a week for their family and not feel guilty about it – not go around apologizing about it or making excuses. Neither my work nor my parenting is perfect, and I'm far from it. But stressing over either takes my energy away without paying it back. I do my best every day and know that tomorrow will offer me another chance to improve."

"I love when my eight-year-old comes home, sits down, does her homework, then says, 'I'm ready to play because I did all my work.' That's what my life is like, I do all my work so I can play."

10

Conclusion

St John of the Cross, a sixteenth century Spanish mystic, wrote that the number one prayer everyone should learn is, *"I am enough"*.

I think we all want to feel like we are enough and that we have enough. Unfortunately, there is a big disconnect between the content of your life and the experience you have of that content. In other words, feeling like you are enough has very little to do with how much you actually have.

We have just examined the stories of people who have changed their lives in some very meaningful and impressive ways. They didn't do this through will power or a quick-fix answer. They did it by using their Thinkers to collaborate with their Emoters to change their Robots, thus changing what was giving rise to the feeling of not having enough. While they did a lot of changing on the outside, the biggest changes happened on the inside.

Our challenge to you, as you work to apply what you've learned in this book, is to keep your eye on the prize: feeling and living like you are enough and have enough.

We sincerely thank you for reading our book, and hope it makes a difference in your life.

Jeff and Jim

About the Authors

Jeff Gaines

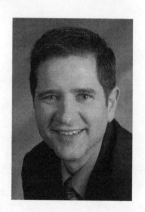

Some have compared the process of writing a book to childbirth. I don't, because I was there when my wife gave birth and I'd rather write a book. Given the things I've had to produce though, this has clearly been at or near the top of the list of the most difficult things I've done.

Why did I do it? Well, it's an obvious choice for someone in my field – that has been part of the motivation, but not all of it, and probably not even most of it. The entire process has caused me to reexamine why I'm in this field in the first place. So, to answer the question of why, let me start with the story of how my career started.

When I was twenty-three years old, I had a high paying job with British Petroleum, was going to school to get an MBA that BP was paying for, owned a nice house, was engaged to be married, and even had a way cool car with tinted windows and leather seats. My friends, my family, my mom – they were soooo proud. Then, in a three-month period, I quit my job, sold my house, dropped out of school, and ended the relationship. I kept the car.

My friends, family, and mom went from being proud to being quite concerned. I was having a mid-twenties crisis. Just like I've heard that fifty is the new thirty and dead is the new eighty, I guess my mid-twenties were the old mid-forties.

When people asked me why I was doing all these things I said, "I don't know what I want but I know I'm not happy, so the way things are now must be wrong." So I trashed everything. It just seemed like everything wasn't enough.

Then I went golfing. I caddied for a semi-pro woman golfer on a small tour in California. I had no idea why – it just seemed like the thing to do. But I wasn't living the carefree life people thought I was. I was a mess: deeply hurting from my ended relationship, confused about my career direction, and pretty much broke.

Then one day, I was talking to a friend who said she was going to take a personal growth course called The Pursuit of Excellence. I had no clue what that meant or what it was about, and neither did she. She just said it looked fun, lasted five days, and cost five hundred dollars. If you didn't like it, they would give you your money back. I thought, "Cool, free seminar," and took it.

It was the first time in my life I had been exposed to any education like it. I think of it as "the knowledge we need to know but don't get taught." The course dealt with topics like: what makes a successful relationship, how to resolve conflicts, persuasion, comfort zones, confidence, and personality types. Today, more and more companies invest in this type of learning.

Skipping forward, I ended up taking several more courses the company offered and entered a program that trained me to be one of their speakers. After a couple of years, I was one of the few who was hired to work for them. At twenty-seven years old, I had the distinction of being one of their youngest facilitators ever – and so I started my new career. That was in 1997 and I've been a speaker in the field of personal and professional growth ever since.

Even bigger than a career change, though, is the new way in which I see the world and approach my life. Before my mid-twenties crisis, I was doing what most people do: get a job, find a good spouse, get a car, maybe have some kids, and then you're happy. But for me, and for many others, the happy part never showed up. While it felt okay, even good, it just didn't seem to be enough.

The basic flaw in my mindset was to think that my experience of life would be determined by the content of my life. It led me to the common way of thinking that as soon as I _____, (finish school, find the right person, have enough money, look the right way, etc.) then I will be happy. When I achieved my goals and the happy part didn't show up, I just figured I had chosen the wrong things or the next thing. I was in the pursuit of happiness through the pursuit of stuff. (With apologies to my ex-fiancé for referring to her as "stuff".)

The big shift in my thinking was to go from living from the outside-in to the inside-out: to recognizing that the only place to pursue happiness is inside my own head. I didn't shave my head and become a Buddhist monk (although those guys seem pretty happy), and I can't say I'm always happy now but I also believe that the expectation of having to be happy all the time is part of what drives the Never Enough mentality in our country.

Since my mid-twenties, I've rebuilt my life with a wonderful wife and son, a great house, great friends, fun stuff to do, and a successful career. To the outside observer, it looks successful, just as it did some twenty years ago. My focus now, however, is not about being happy all the time or wondering what is missing in my life. My life is enough. I actually have more than my fair share, probably more than enough. If I can't find peace and contentment in the life I have, the problem is not with my life.

To answer the original question of why did I write this book, I want you to feel that what you have is enough and who you are is enough. People who feel this way still go after their dreams and work to create more and different aspirations, but not in order to fill some bottomless hole. They do it because life is for living. The most valuable things we accumulate are experiences. Is your experience of life enough?

About the Authors

Jim Sorensen

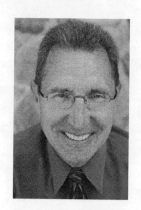

In Jeff's About the Author, he wrote about why he wrote this book. Why I did is very simple: Jeff asked me if I would write it with him. My basic philosophy of life is, if something shows up – it's mine. It is here to either directly benefit me or it's here so that I can benefit someone else. That philosophy has led me to many adventures and, to be quite honest, the benefit often wasn't clear until much later.

In some ways, my story is similar to Jeff's, and very different in other ways. I was raised in a small town in Nebraska on the wrong side of the tracks. I had a draft number of thirty-five, which meant I was going to be drafted. I decided to be smart and enlist in the Navy because logically (from a Nebraska mindset), the closest I would ever be to the war in Vietnam would be miles offshore. Little did I know about the brown water Navy. I spent the next three years of my young life on the Mekong River. There are many bad things about war but one great thing is that it woke me up. I noticed a whole world out there, full of new experiences, new people, and new adventures galore.

After the war, my adventures continued and included being married twice (each lasting less than a year) and having lots of other short-term relationships. I also had many short-term jobs, including owning a retail craft store and becoming a Scrimshander (ivory carver). I traveled around the country doing scrimshaw demonstrations and real estate marketing and a couple of other things. I was a great starter. I loved the excitement of the new but didn't know what to do after that.

Like Jeff, I took a class that woke me up. As a result, I still love new adventures but I've found ways to fulfill that desire more constructively. I've now been designing and leading classes for thirty-three years, and have been with my wife for twenty-seven years (best decision I've ever made). A couple of years ago, someone told me that he respected me for my commitment to my marriage. I replied, "I'm not committed to my marriage." He looked extremely surprised. I said, "I'm committed to the quality of my marriage." I'm not good at forcing myself to do anything, so my whole focus is to make sure my relationship and my career are so good that I'd be a fool to leave. So far, so good.

The part that I really enjoyed about this process was the collaboration. There is something about noodling on something interesting with someone I respect that is one of my greatest pleasures in life.

For Your Business

This book is designed to be about your entire life, not just work, and not just personal. However, Jim and I hope that you can see how this content would benefit a company or organization, especially since that is where you likely spend a significant portion of your life.

We are both speakers and consultants to the business world, and hope you'll consider how we might benefit your organization. The framework of this book, the three drivers of the Internal Game and the Robot Reprogramming Formula, can be applied to any area. Here, we focused specifically on health, wealth, and stress. When giving keynotes or workshops, we focus on areas such as sales, customer service, management, leadership, communication, motivation, team building, and more.

To learn more about our offerings for the business world, check out our corporate site:

TheInternalGame.com

Give us a call. We'd love to work with you and your organization.

18375602R00116

Made in the USA
Charleston, SC
31 March 2013